Succeeding in Your Medical Degree

Titles in the Series

Professional Practice for Foundation Doctors ISBN 9780857252845
Health, Behaviour and Society: a Companion to Clinical Medicine ISBN 9780857254610
Law and Ethics in Medical Practice ISBN 9780857250988

To order, please contact our distributor: BEBC Distribution, Albion Close, Parkstone, Poole, BH12 3LL. Telephone: 0845 230 9000, email: learningmatters@bebc.co.uk.
You can also find more information on each of these titles and our other learning resources at www.learningmatters.co.uk

Succeeding in Your Medical Degree

Editor: Simon Watmough

Series Editors:

Judy McKimm, Kirsty Forrest and Aidan Byrne

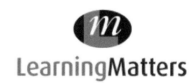

First published in 2011 by Learning Matters Ltd

British Library Cataloguing in Publication Data
A CIP record for this book is available from the British Library.
ISBN 978 0 85725 397 2

This book is also available in the following formats:
Adobe ebook ISBN: 978 0 85725 399 6
EPUB ebook ISBN: 978 0 85725 398 9
Kindle ISBN: 978 0 85725 400 9

Cover and text design by Code 5 Design Associates
Project management by Swales & Willis Ltd, Exeter, Devon
Typeset by Swales & Willis Ltd, Exeter, Devon
Printed and bound in Great Britain by Short Run Press Ltd, Exeter, Devon

Learning Matters Ltd
20 Cathedral Yard
Exeter EX1 1HB
Tel: 01392 215560
info@learningmatters.co.uk
www.learningmatters.co.uk

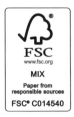

FSC
www.fsc.org
MIX
Paper from
responsible sources
FSC® C014540

Contents

Contents

Foreword from the Series Editors

The Learning Matters Medical Education Series

Medical education is currently experiencing yet another a period of change typified in the UK with the introduction of the revised *Tomorrow's Doctors* (General Medical Council, 2009) and ongoing work on establishing core curricula for many subject areas. This new series of textbooks has been developed as a direct response to these changes and the impact on undergraduate medical education.

Research indicates that effective medical practitioners combine excellent, up-to-date clinical and scientific knowledge with practical skills and the ability to work with patients, families and other professionals with empathy and understanding, they know when to lead and when to follow and they work collaboratively and professionally to improve health outcomes for individuals and communities. The General Medical Council has defined a series of learning outcomes set out under three headings:

- Doctor as Practitioner

- Doctor as Scholar and Scientist

- Doctor as Professional

The books in this series do not cover practical clinical procedures or knowledge about diseases and conditions, but instead cover the range of non-technical professional skills (plus underpinning knowledge) that students and doctors need to know in order to become effective, safe and competent practitioners.

Aimed specifically at medical students (but also of use for junior doctors, teachers and clinicians), each book relates to specific outcomes of *Tomorrow's Doctors*, providing both knowledge and help to improve the skills necessary to be successful at the non-clinical aspects of training as a doctor. One of the aims of the series is to set medical practice within the wider social, policy and organisational agendas to help produce future doctors who are socially aware and willing and prepared to engage in broader issues relating to healthcare delivery.

Individual books in the series outline the key theoretical approaches and policy agendas relevant to that subject, and go further by demonstrating through case studies and scenarios how these theories can be used in work settings to achieve best practice. Plenty of activities and self-assessment tools throughout the book will help the reader to hone their critical thinking and reflection skills.

Chapters in each of the books follow a standard format. At the beginning a box highlights links to relevant competencies and outcomes from *Tomorrow's Doctors* and other medical curricula if appropriate. This sets the scene and enables the reader to see exactly what will be covered. This is extended by a chapter overview which sets out the key topics and what the student should expect to have learnt by the end of the chapter.

There is at least one case study in each chapter which considers how theory can be used in practice from different perspectives. Activities are included which include practical tasks with learning points, critical thinking research tasks and reflective practice/thinking points. Activities can be carried out by the reader or with others and are designed to raise awareness, consolidate understanding of theories and ideas and enable the student to improve their practice by using models, approaches and ideas. Each activity is followed by a brief discussion on issues raised. At the end of each chapter a chapter summary provides an aide-memoire of what has been covered.

All chapters are evidence based in that they set out the theories or evidence that underpins practice. In most chapters, one or more 'What's the evidence' boxes provide further information about a particular piece of research or a policy agenda through books, articles, websites or policy papers. A list of additional readings is set out under the 'Going further' section, with all references collated at the end of the book.

The series is edited by Professor Judy McKimm, Dr Kirsty Forrest and Dr Aidan Byrne, all of whom are experienced medical educators and writers. Book and chapter authors are drawn from a wide pool of practising clinicians and educators from the UK and internationally.

Author Biographies

Andrew Bowhay

Andrew is a consultant paediatric anaesthetist with an interest in both undergraduate and post-graduate medical education. Currently one of his educational roles is as an associate postgraduate dean in the Mersey Deanery. Andrew has also been a clinical sub dean for undergraduate medical training at his hospital as well as the clinical strategist for the Centre for Excellence in Teaching and Learning at the University of Liverpool. Andrew has undertaken research on trainees' attitudes to the European Working Time Directive and how well medical schools perform in postgraduate medical examinations. Andrew is also an undergraduate and postgraduate examiner with a particular interest in standard setting.

Gemma Cherry

Gemma is a research assistant within the School of Medicine at the University of Liverpool, where she is studying for a PhD looking at the relationship between emotional intelligence and empathetic communication style in medical students and foundation doctors. She also works part time as a reviewer of clinical evidence at the Liverpool Reviews and Implementation Group (LRIG), which produces systematic reviews of clinical and cost effectiveness of treatments/drugs for the National Institute of Clinical Excellence.

Ray Fewtrell

Ray is currently a research fellow in the School of Medicine at the University of Liverpool. He spent the last 14 years researching the portfolios, critical thinking, reflection and assessment within under-graduate medical students. He supervises medical students on student selected components from years 1 to 3, is co-lead on the professional reflective document, has been a problem-based learning facilitator, admission interviewer, personal tutor and an examiner at OSCEs. He currently sits on the SSC moderating board, clinical team and clinical programme committees.

Jayne Garner

Jayne is currently working as a research associate in the Department for Health Services Research at the University of Liverpool. She obtained a degree in sociology and a master's degree in social research methods from the University of Northumbria. She worked in local government for eight years in policy development, consultation and community engagement before joining the University of Liverpool in 2007 to study for a PhD in medical education. Jayne has also been a problem-based learning convener, an examiner at OSCEs and a personal tutor.

Michael Moneypenny

Michael Moneypenny read biochemistry at the University of Bath and Medicine at the University of Dundee. He is a specialist registrar in anaesthesia and an honorary lecturer at the University of Liverpool. His research interests concentrate on medical education, simulation and the impact of human factors on patient safety. Dr Moneypenny is currently evaluating a tool for assessing team work and leadership skills.

Helen O'Sullivan

Helen O'Sullivan is the director of the Centre for Excellence in Excellence Based Learning and Teaching in the Faculty of Health and Life Sciences, University of Liverpool where she works across the Faculty on areas such as curriculum development and learning and teaching. As the director of the School of Medicine's CETL for four years, she led research and teaching in developing professionalism in medical undergraduates. She is particularly interested in investigating methods for assessing attitudes and behaviour and in the role emotional intelligence plays in professionalism and medical leadership.

Dan Robinson

Dan currently manages the e-learning provision for the School of Medicine at the University of Liverpool and is also a member of the Centre for Excellence in Evidence-Based Learning and Teaching. Having 13 years' experience in the field, he now provides a strategic direction and recently took the leading role in writing the first 'Technology Enhanced Learning' strategy for the school. Dan is now in the implementation stages of this strategy and is heavily involved in a project to develop a management framework to underpin future e-learning developments. He is also involved in e-assessment at university level and is a member of the Association for Learning Technologists.

Christine Waddelove

Christine is currently employed as a senior careers adviser at the University of Liverpool developing and delivering career planning and guidance programmes for undergraduate medical students. She also teaches medical students on student selected components from years 1 to 3 where students complete an SSC on a 'careers' related area. She is also involved in offering careers advice and guidance to medical students on an individual basis as well as organising careers events. She works closely with a number of other external organisations including the Association of Graduate Careers Advisory Service (AGCAS), the Institute of Careers Guidance (ICG), UKFPO and Mersey Deanery. She hopes in her work to inspire students to explore their career aspirations and consider their wider career management skills and interests while at medical school.

Simon Watmough

Simon is currently a research fellow in medical education at the University of Liverpool. He has spent the last ten years researching the content and influence of undergraduate medical curricula from the perspective of students, junior doctors and senior doctors. He has researched the impact of *Tomorrow's Doctors* on UK medical education and has a PhD in medical education. He also teaches medical students on student selected components from years 1 to 4, has been a problem-based learning convener, an examiner at objective structured clinical examinations (OSCEs) and sits on the special study module moderating board.

At the time of writing all authors of this book were members of the Centre of Excellence for Developing Professionalism, School of Medicine, University of Liverpool.

Introduction

This book will examine some of the key themes in undergraduate medical education today that run across undergraduate curricula in the UK. Medical students across different institutions will assume they will learn about the clinical sciences, such as anatomy, physiology and pathology and disease processes, but there is more to medical education than just learning the science relevant to becoming a doctor today. Learning about sciences is covered in many other textbooks so this book will focus on the themes inherent across all undergraduate courses outside the sciences which students may not be aware of, but are just as important for becoming a good doctor.

We will be referring throughout to *Tomorrow's Doctors* (GMC, 2009a), a revised and updated version of a document first published in 1993 by the General Medical Council (GMC). This includes the latest guidelines on undergraduate medical education to which all medical schools in the UK must adhere. The first version of *Tomorrow's Doctors* (GMC, 1993) had a marked impact on medical education in the UK, as Chapters 1 and 2 will make clear.

In this book we give a brief history of medical education in the UK, why *Tomorrow's Doctors* was written and the evidence behind it. We outline some of the key themes from these recommendations, and examine the implications both for the content of medical curricula and for students embarking on a medical degree and their careers after graduation. *Tomorrow's Doctors* refers to and incorporates elements of other GMC publications such as *The New Doctor* and *Good Medical Practice*, and these are cited throughout the book where relevant.

Our book is aimed primarily as a guide for medical students. However, it will also be useful for all medical educators, both clinical and non-clinical and for students considering undertaking a medical degree. It shows why medical curricula in the UK look the way they do today and discusses some of the most important themes in medical education. This book also suggests ways to get the best out of your undergraduate medical education and the relevance of this education after graduation when students become doctors. It gives key references as a base to explore the literature, shows what the current evidence is surrounding each of the themes in the book, provides activities to follow which will make the reader think about each theme and includes case studies that illuminate each theme of the book.

Book structure

Chapter 1 looks at the role of the GMC in UK medical education and how this has developed historically. There is also a discussion about the other influences on undergraduate medical education, such as the Quality Assurance Agency and EU directives. It looks at historical recommendations on medical education and how a stage was reached in 1993 when the GMC felt it had to issue radical recommendations on UK undergraduate medical education and how the 2009 *Tomorrow's Doctors* will affect UK students over the next few years.

Chapter 2 summarises the original *Tomorrow's Doctors* and the most recent revision and highlights how it has changed since 1993. It also outlines some of the research projects that have evaluated the document and the evidence that has informed the latest version.

Chapter 3 outlines what medical professionalism is, why it has recently come to prominence in UK medical education and why the GMC places such an emphasis on it in its latest documents. It also examines why it is important for doctors to be professional and how you can develop professionalism from an early stage.

Chapter 4 explains why doctors need leadership training and how leadership will be an important part of your working life. The chapter will discuss whether all doctors need to be managers and leaders and what opportunities there are to develop leadership skills as undergraduates.

Chapter 5 explains the different types of assessment that you are likely to undergo, including knowledge-based, practical and continuous assessment and the theory behind them and how pass marks are established. It also explores ways you can improve your performances through feedback and understanding exams.

Chapter 6 addresses the important issue of communication skills and, specifically, factors associated with effective communication in medicine. It also provides a summary of the core components of communication skills teaching programmes in undergraduate medical education. Finally, it examines the value of various teaching methods, such as role play, feedback and video analysis, in the acquisition of effective communication skills.

Chapter 7 explores why simulation is being used today in medical education. It discusses the strengths and weaknesses of the different types of simulation used and how embracing simulation can help students to be successful at medical school and to become good doctors.

Chapter 8 shows how important student selected components (SSCs) are to developing the skills that all doctors will need once they graduate. It also shows that they can be interesting and fun and offers advice on how to get the most out of an elective period.

Chapter 9 demonstrates how peer feedback (including peer review, peer appraisal and peer assessment) is a key challenge for students but can be invaluable in gaining advice about how to improve performance and gain the generic skills needed to be a doctor.

Chapter 10 takes you through what to expect from and how to get the most out of what many see as the most important part of medical education – clinical placements. It outlines the different ways students learn in both the community and in hospital specialities and how they develop communication skills, history and examination and practical skills on clinical placements.

Chapter 11 discusses why medical careers are such a big topic in medical education today. It gives practical advice on how to make the most of undergraduate education to prepare for postgraduate decision making and how to develop strategies to make students more employable after graduation.

Chapter 12 shows how effective management of information is important in many aspects of health practice from recording patient contact, communicating and managing personal and professional development, to helping students succeed at medical school and then as a junior doctor. It shows how to develop information technology (IT) skills and how these skills can help the student to become a reflective practitioner.

Chapter 13 is the concluding chapter in which we summarise the book and speculate about the way medical education may evolve in future years.

We hope that you find this book stimulating and enjoyable and we encourage you to take advantage of the wide range of activities and case studies that each chapter offers, helping you to understand theory and more importantly relating it to your practice.

chapter 1

The Role of the General Medical Council in UK Medical Education

Simon Watmough

Introduction

You will have heard of the General Medical Council (GMC) as you embark on your undergraduate degree in the UK. The GMC is frequently in the news, although this is often regarding disciplinary action against practising doctors, so some of you may think that the GMC is only relevant to qualified doctors. However, all UK undergraduate medical curricula have to conform to the recommendations made by the GMC on undergraduate medical education in their *Tomorrow's Doctors* documents and medical schools have a statutory duty to prepare graduates to work and train as junior doctors in accordance with these GMC guidelines. This chapter will give a brief history of medical education in the UK, examining the role of the GMC in UK medical education and discussing why *Tomorrow's Doctors* was written and the evidence behind it.

The role of the GMC in undergraduate medical education

The GMC is the regulatory body for medicine and medical education in the UK and has a statutory duty set out by law to set standards for medical education and decide who is fit to be a doctor registered with the GMC. No one in the UK can legally practise medicine unless they are on the GMC register. Although medical schools and undergraduate curricula in the UK are diverse and there is no 'common curriculum' by which all medical schools are guided, they are all required to comply with the recommendations issued by the GMC Education Committee.

There has been some kind of regulation in medicine and medical education in Britain for a long time. For example, in 1421 Parliament petitioned Henry V to pass a law determining that a medicine degree from a university was the only qualification granting the right to practise. In 1462 Edward IV gave a charter to the Company of Barbers allowing them to carry out surgery. In 1511 Henry VIII decreed that no person should practise as physician or surgeon within the City of London unless examined and approved by the Bishop of London or a Dean of St Paul's Cathedral.

By the nineteenth century there were many different bodies regulating the medical profession and they all had different standards and interests. Prior to 1858 there were 19 separate licensing bodies in operation throughout the UK and none of them had a national jurisdiction. For example, an Edinburgh practitioner might not be able to practise legally in London or even Glasgow. In the mid-nineteenth century there were still a large number of charlatans, quacks, teeth pullers and bone setters with little formal training. There was a huge chasm between the 'charlatans' and those students who learned medicine, often at a great cost, through the universities or corporations, who inevitably felt cheated out of their educational investment (Stacey, 1992). As a result of this an Act of Parliament was passed in 1858 called The Medical Act, which established a national system of regulating medicine and medical education by creating the General Medical Council. The Act gave the GMC power to hold a register of practitioners and to set the standard for entrance to the profession by controlling the standards of medical education, and the GMC was made directly responsible to the Privy Council.

The GMC began to exercise its powers over medical education soon after the Act was passed. In 1867 the Council decided on the ten medical subjects that should be obligatory in terms of undergraduate teaching and examination: descriptive and general anatomy; physiology; chemistry; material medica; practical pharmacy; medicine; surgery; midwifery and forensic medicine. It was notable that that there was nothing in terms of communication skills, professionalism or practical skills! The first committee was made up of representatives of medical corporations, universities, colleges and six independent members nominated by the Crown. The GMC had the power to ask schools for information about current courses of study and the examinations. They did not have the power to stipulate a compulsory curriculum, just to say 'sufficient' or 'insufficient' regarding individual courses.

From 1867 to 1993 medical education and the content of undergraduate medical education largely followed similar patterns at universities. The first half of medical degrees involved intensive, didactic lectures in the sciences followed by clinical placements towards the end of the course so there were distinct preclinical and clinical sections. There was little, if any, formal communication or clinical skills training, few opportunities to experience general practice or opportunities to study topics that interested students in-depth. The publication of *Tomorrow's Doctors*, however, was to bring about a major change in medical education and explains why the content of your medical curriculum looks as it does today.

ACTIVITY 1.1

Take a look at the GMC website and look at their role today. Search the internet for other regulatory bodies that regulate medical education elsewhere in the world. What similarities do you see between them?

Why reform undergraduate medical curricula?

There were a series of international pressures influencing medical education in the UK by the early 1990s. The World Federation for Medical Education (WFME) issued the Edinburgh Declaration of 12 principles for reforming medical education in 1988 (Parsell and Bligh, 1995). Also, many medical schools around the world, but in particular in North America, had radically altered their curricula with seemingly very few adverse effects (Albanese and Mitchell, 1993). For example, major reform with the introduction of problem-based learning (PBL) took place at McMaster University in Canada in 1962 and spread in the 1970s to other schools further afield, such as the University of Maastricht medical school (The Netherlands) and the University of Newcastle (Australia), so there were already precedents from outside the UK on managing curriculum reform away from traditional curricula.

There was also a growing feeling that too much 'irrelevant' knowledge was being taught to undergraduates and that in the preclinical part of the course students were learning biochemistry, anatomy and physiology which they would not need in their work as doctors. Having distinct clinical and preclinical sections to medical curricula seemed to exacerbate this and it was not always clear which was the most relevant knowledge for clinical practice.

Critics had been arguing for many years about the content of medical curricula and the didactic nature of medical education. Richard Davis wrote about the problem of excessive anatomy lectures in the 1750s. William Barrett Marshall, a student in the 1820s, felt the factual burden on students should be reduced and that thinking and reasoning should be encouraged instead. He also suggested that students should learn integrated anatomy teaching, long before it was introduced into UK medical curricula. In 1835 the *London Gazette* wrote that students should learn about public and private hygiene at the expense of pathology (Poynter, 1966). The opening pages of the original *Tomorrow's Doctors* states that well over 100 years ago there were significant concerns that student doctors were not being given enough time for self-education and that there was far too much emphasis on gaining knowledge in medical curricula. The document quotes from Thomas Huxley in 1876:

The burden we place on the medical student is far too heavy, and it takes some doing to keep from breaking his intellectual back. A system of medical education that is actually calculated to obstruct the acquisition of sound knowledge and to heavily favour the crammer and grinder is a disgrace.

By the late twentieth century this was widely seen as being at the expense of learning the skills to work as a junior doctor.

ACTIVITY 1.2

- Why do you think it is important to have a regulator in medical education?
- Do you think medical education would be better or worse without a regulator?
- Do you think that regulation of undergraduate medical education will automatically lead to better doctors?

Medical education from 1945 to *Tomorrow's Doctors*

After the Second World War and the introduction of the National Health Service (NHS) there were a series of Acts of Parliament and recommendations from the GMC which had further impact on undergraduate medical education and led directly to the publication of the original *Tomorrow's Doctors*. The introduction of a preregistration year in 1953 was crucial to the development of undergraduate medical education as much as postgraduate medical education. The preregistration year was a direct result of the Goodenough Report (Goodenough, 1944) which for the first time recognised the need for further, supervised training after the undergraduate degree. The report also recommended provision for an increase in student numbers to produce extra doctors for the NHS which was introduced in 1948. The fact that the report recommended a preregistration year to ease the burden on undergraduate curricula highlighted the concerns even then about the preparedness of junior doctors for practice after graduation.

In 1957, the GMC (1957) advised a 'lighter and more flexible' curriculum, asking medical schools to consider experimenting with curriculum content and teaching methods. In 1962 the Porritt Report (Porritt, 1962) concluded 'We cannot escape the conclusion that the medical facilities of British Universities are now lagging considerably behind those of many comparable countries in respect of research facilities, accommodation and available teachers.' It also pointed out that students seemed to have a narrow experience of the range of clinical work with a lack of exposure to community medicine.

Before 1972, Parliament largely left the GMC to its own devices but a 'revolt' in the late 1960s over compulsory payments to enter the medical register forced Parliament to take a closer interest into the role and function of the GMC. As a result the Merrison Inquiry was set up to look at how the GMC was operating at that time. One of the recommendations of the Inquiry suggested that the GMC had to raise the standard of undergraduate and postgraduate education 'to make a clinician out of the graduate' (Merrison Report, 1975). Merrison also commented on what he saw as the failure of the educational component of the preregistration year. The Merrison Report was a big influence on the 1978 and then 1983 Medical Acts, which officially recognised that the aim of undergraduate medical education was no longer to produce a graduate who was competent in medicine, surgery and obstetrics (as it had been since the nineteenth century) but rather to create graduates capable of going onto postgraduate training and able to work as junior doctors.

Crucially, the 1978 Act reformed the structure of the GMC and created a semi-independent education committee, stating that the GMC should be responsible for co-ordinating all stages of medical education and promoting high standards. The Education Committee was given extended powers to visit universities and more control over the preregistration year. In the early 1980s the Education Committee started using its rights to visit medical schools to see how its recommendations of 1980 were being implemented. There was some anxiety about interfering in 'university autonomy' (Stacey, 1992) and at first only qualified doctors were included in the visiting parties. This set a precedent for more thorough visits which started in the 1990s following the publication of *Tomorrow's Doctors*. As the 1990s approached, the GMC was taking a more active interest in undergraduate medical education which was indicated by making regular formal visits to medical schools.

The under-utilisation of general practice in undergraduate medical education was also contributing to the problems in medical education (Bligh and Parsell, 1995).

By the 1990s over 90 per cent of NHS consultations took place in the community, yet many medical schools only had token short placements in general practice in their curriculum. Many generic medical skills could be learned in the community and it was suggested that this would also help students gain more of an insight into the social and emotional factors involved in medicine. There was a belief among medical educators in the need to include more public health medicine to enable doctors to deal with infectious diseases such as HIV or TB; a shift in emphasis from hospital care to community care; a greater sharing of care within multiprofessional teams; an ageing, multiracial society; new sciences and techniques in medicine; increasing public expectations and the need for doctors to include patients in the treatment process (Bullimore, 1998).

The public view of doctors had changed and people were often less willing to be sympathetic to the actions of doctors or to take what they said at face value. Patients expected their doctors to have good communication skills and to include them in the treatment process. Finally, there was overwhelming evidence by the 1990s that many doctors felt inadequately prepared to work as junior doctors as a result of undergraduate training (GMC, 1993).

By the 1990s the GMC wanted doctors who were capable of independent learning and critical thought (Fraser, 1991) and who had the ability to cope with change, which was essential in the professional environment (Irvine, 1993). But the medical education available at that time was not seen as delivering this. An important study by Calman and Donaldson (1991) concluded that UK medical graduates were not being prepared to work as junior doctors. By 1993 there was overwhelming evidence that further reform was necessary.

Other GMC and EU documents on medical education

UK medical schools are also required to conform to directives on undergraduate medical education from the European Union (EU) and to the Quality Assurance Agency (QAA) guidelines. The QAA's role is to safeguard the public interest in higher education degrees and encourage improvement in the UK (QAA, 2010). The QAA has visited UK medical schools and published details of their visits on their website. The EU stipulates how many hours of undergraduate studies doctors should have and how many hours they can work when training as junior doctors. Therefore, a number of bodies regulate and influence the content and length of your medical education.

Medical schools and doctors at various stages of their career have to be aware of other GMC publications such as *The New Doctor*, first published in 1997 and updated in 2009. It illustrates in detail what newly qualified doctors should be able to undertake and what they should be learning. As the aim of the undergraduate medical education in the UK is to produce graduates capable of working and training as junior doctors, there is considerable overlap between these two documents. The GMC produces online guidance and documents for all practising doctors including *Good Medical Practice* (GMC, 2006), which includes their definition of 'Duties of a doctor' showing the standards to which doctors should aspire. Again, these are useful guides for medical students who will become doctors after they graduate (GMC, 2006).

The GMC website also includes guidance and case examples on a wide range of topics including ethics and law, health and wellbeing, professionalism and management.

ACTIVITY 1.3

Search the internet or look in your medical school common room or library for the GMC's guidelines in *The New Doctor* and *Good Medical Practice* and guidance on 'Duties of a doctor'. What similarities do you see between the themes in these documents and *Tomorrow's Doctors*?

GMC visits to medical schools

The GMC now visits medical schools at least twice within a 10-year period to see whether they are conforming to the required standards and *Tomorrow's Doctors* and it publishes the results of these visits on the GMC website. In addition, all new schools or programmes are visited throughout the first run through of the programme until students are in their foundation programme. These visits are made by teams working under the QABME (Quality Assurance of Basic Medical Education) process. These teams include clinician members of the GMC Education Committee, lay members, other health care professionals and representatives from other medical schools. The teams consider documentation, study assessment procedures, visit training facilities such as clinical skills and anatomy resource centres, hospital sites and lecture theatres and interview staff and students.

ACTIVITY 1.4

Look on the GMC website for details of their last visit to your medical school. What did they say was good about your curriculum? What did they say could be improved?

Chapter summary

- Medical schools in the UK have to conform with the expectations of a range of regulatory and statutory bodies, including the GMC, QAA and EU.

- There was overwhelming evidence that reform in medical education was needed prior to 1993 when the GMC introduced *Tomorrow's Doctors*, its recommendations on undergraduate medical education.

- *Tomorrow's Doctors* heralded major reform in UK medical education which has been followed by a series of ongoing educational reforms and curriculum change aimed primarily at improving the competence of graduating students.

GOING FURTHER

- Parsell, G and Bligh, J (1995) The changing context of undergraduate medical education. *Postgraduate Medical Journal*, 71: 394–403.

- Bullimore, D (1998) *Study Skills and Tomorrow's Doctors*. London: WB Saunders.

- Calman, K and Donaldson, M (1991) The pre-registration house officer year: a critical incident study. *Medical Education*, 25: 51–59.

- Fraser, R (1991) Undergraduate medical education: present state and future needs. *British Medical Journal*, 303: 41–43.

- General Medical Council (1991) *Undergraduate Medical Education: The Need for Change*. London: GMC.

These articles/books discuss the state of medical education pre-1993 and help show why a stage was reached where reform of UK undergraduate medical education was required.

chapter 2

Tomorrow's Doctors and **Medical Education**
Simon Watmough

Chapter overview

This chapter will outline the key recommendations contained in the first edition of *Tomorrow's Doctors* (GMC, 1993). It will show how the UK moved away from traditional medical curricula in the 1990s, summarise the recommendations in the latest version and show how they have affected the content of undergraduate medical curricula in the UK while exploring the similarities and differences between the two documents. Understanding these two versions of *Tomorrow's Doctors* will help you gain the most out of the tips and advice contained in the rest of this book and your undergraduate medical education.

The original *Tomorrow's Doctors* (1993)

The document emphasises throughout that students should be prepared to work and train as first year medical graduates, not specialists, thus making the preparation for the first postgraduate year the central outcome of undergraduate medical education, reinforcing the recommendations of the 1983 Medical Act (see Chapter 1).

As Chapter 1 highlights, throughout *Tomorrow's Doctors* (GMC, 1993) many references are made to reducing the 'factual burden' and discussing the 'gross overcrowding' in undergraduate curricula and that 'the scarcely tolerable burden of information that is imposed taxes the memory and not the intellect. The emphasis is on the passive acquisition of knowledge, much of it to become outdated or forgotten.' It also suggests that a way round this would be to integrate the science and clinical teaching in the core curriculum so that the undergraduate curriculum is the 'first step in the continuum of medical education'. With a structure of specialist training in place, the document recognises there was a case for moving some factual knowledge to a later stage of medical training. The GMC called for 'essential' knowledge to be covered by the 'core curriculum' and suggested that each 'core curriculum' should be freely available so medical schools are aware of the content of each other's curricula.

According to *Tomorrow's Doctors*, medical students should also learn about evidence-based understanding of diagnosis and diseases while making the most of modern information technology. Assessment procedures should reflect these aims and there should be a movement away from, for example, multiple choice questions to a system that encourages certification of achievement in competency and reduces emphasis on the uncritical acquisition of facts. The GMC document suggested that multiple choice format tends to 'put a premium on the acquisition of facts at the expense of reasoning'. It also called for improvement in clinical skills teaching and assessment, including better experience of undertaking practical skills, and that students should be formally assessed on these skills prior to graduation in order to ensure they have the required skills to work as first year graduates. It also recommended the increased use of logbooks or computer-based systems for recording student experience and performance in place of 'traditional' exams.

The key points of *Tomorrow's Doctors*

The key themes of the original *Tomorrow's Doctors* are as follows:

- Attitudes and behaviour that are suitable for a doctor must be developed. Students must develop qualities that are appropriate to their future responsibilities to patients, colleagues and society in general.

- The core curriculum must set out the essential knowledge, skills and attitudes students should have by the time they graduate.

- The core curriculum must be supported by a series of student-selected components that allow students to study, in depth, areas of particular interest to them.

- The core curriculum must be the responsibility of clinicians, basic scientists and medical educationalists working together to integrate their contributions and achieve a common purpose.

- Factual information must be kept to the essential minimum that students need at this stage of medical education.

- Learning opportunities must help students to explore knowledge, and evaluate and integrate (bring together) evidence critically. The curriculum must motivate students and help them develop the skills for self-directed learning.

- The essential skills that graduates need must be gained under supervision. Medical schools must assess students' competence in these skills.

- The curriculum must stress the importance of communication skills and the other essential skills of medical practice.

- The health and safety of the public must be an important part of the curriculum.

- Clinical education must reflect the changing patterns of health care and provide experience in a variety of clinical settings.

- Teaching and learning systems must take account of modern educational theory and research, and make use of modern technologies where evidence shows that these are effective.

- Schemes of assessment must take account of best practice, support the curriculum, make sure that the intended curricular outcomes are assessed and reward performance appropriately

- When designing a curriculum, putting it into practice and continually reviewing it, medical schools must set up effective supervisory structures that use an appropriate range of expertise and knowledge.

The GMC also set out to encourage student choice outside the core curriculum and argued for special study modules or student selected components (SSCs) to facilitate this, which should also encourage critical thinking and develop lifelong learning skills, which of course could be reinforced by the introduction of problem-based learning (PBL) into the curriculum. PBL was also envisaged as a way of reducing the 'factual burden' of teaching unnecessary didactic science knowledge through the lectures which were used in traditional curricula and would reduce the capacity of individual departments to 'overload' the curriculum. Only a minority of medical schools in the UK have introduced PBL but all have modified their science teaching in the last few years and have seen a reduction in the amount of lectures. Many medical schools still use lectures; some use lectures with PBL, others use lectures with small group discussion, case-based teaching, practical sessions in the laboratories or use SSCs so that students can research science areas that interest them. For example, a student thinking about a career in surgery may choose to undertake a number of SSCs in anatomy (see Chapter 8 for more details on SSCs).

ACTIVITY 2.1

All UK medical schools have an outline of their curriculum on their website. Look at the curricula of three different medical schools in the UK, including one of the problem-based learning medical schools. What similarities and what differences do you see? How different are they from the traditional preclinical/clinical curricula of 20 or 30 years ago? What do you think are the strengths and weaknesses of each curriculum in meeting the aims of the GMC?

Tomorrow's Doctors 1993 also stipulated that medical schools should demonstrate to the student the importance of legal and ethical issues, cultural social and emotional and psychological problems and impact of illness on the patients' family. Allied to this is a need to understand health promotion, disease prevention and knowledge of public health and tied in with these was the need to recognise the effects of an ageing population. The GMC also recognised that the public had changing aspirations and called for improvement in practical skills training.

The document also highlighted the attitudinal objectives of undergraduate medical education, including: showing respect for patients and colleagues; being aware of limitations; knowing when to ask for help and being aware of limitations and coping with uncertainty. Students were expected to participate in the peer review and keep a record of their own skills and be aware of their own professional development needs. *Tomorrow's Doctors* called for doctors to be educated with an understanding of other health care professionals and primary care. Clinical teaching should reflect the changing patterns of health care so there should be greater experience of primary care alongside hospital teaching, which would help all students gain a greater understanding of the social and emotional factors in medicine as highlighted in Chapter 1. These recommendations were set out in the postgraduate setting in the 1997 document *The New Doctor* (GMC, 1997), which clarified the skills and competencies expected of UK graduates in the first postgraduate year.

Case study: The University of Liverpool Medical Curriculum before and after *Tomorrow's Doctors*

In 1996 the University of Liverpool introduced a new curriculum based on the recommendations in *Tomorrow's Doctors*. Prior to 1996, Liverpool had a very traditional, lecture-based curriculum which comprised a five-term preclinical course followed by a nine-term clinical course with little formal integration between the two parts of the curriculum. In the first five terms students undertook an intensive series of lectures and practicals in biochemistry, biology, biostatistics, genetics, anatomy, physiology, psychology and pathology. Students then had lectures and clinical placements in separate blocks in general medicine (including care for the elderly), general surgery (including orthopaedics), obstetrics and gynaecology (O & G), psychiatry, ear, nose and throat (ENT), child health, dermatology, cardiology, ophthalmology, neurology, haematology, pharmacology and a three-week placement in general practice. Examinations took place during both sections of the course culminating in final exams at the end of the fifth year in medicine, surgery and O & G. There were no formal communication or clinical skills classes.

In 1996 problem-based learning replaced lectures as the main learning tool in the first four years of the course. Supported by plenary sessions, online resources and a Human Anatomy Resource Centre (HARC), students now develop their own learning objectives during PBL tutorials. Science teaching is integrated throughout the course with clinical exposure increasing each year. Practical and clinical skills are taught in the University's Clinical Skills Resource Centre from the first semester and in hospital centres in later years of the course. Student selected components in the form of special study modules account for approximately 25 per cent of the course and 25 per cent of clinical attachments take place in the community and general practice. Students attend clinical skills classes in the early years of the course and are assessed on all clinical skills throughout the course.

The final year is an apprentice year designed to prepare students to work as postgraduates and includes a 'shadow' placement, general practice and accident and emergency (A & E) placement and two placements in clinical specialties which they choose themselves. Final exams take place at the end of the fourth year and the fifth and final year assessments comprise portfolio and Professional Education and Training Appraisal (PETA) interviews.

What's the evidence?

The following papers show some of the results from work which has evaluated the impact on the competencies of graduates on recommendations of the 1993 *Tomorrow's Doctors*.

These papers show that students who have graduated from medical curricula based on the recommendation of *Tomorrow's Doctors* are better prepared for the practical aspects of working as junior doctors.

O'Neill, P, Willis, S and Jones, A (2003) Does a new undergraduate curriculum based on *Tomorrow's Doctors* prepare house officers better for their first post? A qualitative study of the views of pre-registration house officers using critical incidents. *Medical Education*, 37: 1100–1108.

Watmough, S, Ryland, I, Garden, A and Taylor, D (2006a) Educational supervisors' views on the competencies of pre registration house officers. *British Journal of Hospital Medicine*, 67: 638–664.

Watmough, S, Ryland, I, Taylor, D and Garden, A (2006b) Pre-registration house officer skills and competency assessment through questionnaires. *British Journal of Hospital Medicine*, 67: 487–490.

Tomorrow's Doctors (2009)

Another version of *Tomorrow's Doctors* was published in 2003, which updated the 1993 document and contained similar themes and recommendations to the first document. The 2003 and 2009 versions are set out differently from the first version; the first version goes into more detail about why the GMC are setting out their recommendations whereas the later versions concentrate on the recommendations themselves.

In 2007 the GMC commissioned research into the preparedness of medical graduates to begin practice to inform the 2009 *Tomorrow's Doctors*. This work was undertaken by the Northern Deanery and the Universities of Newcastle, Warwick and Glasgow (Illing *et al.*, 2008). The work included interviewing graduates from all three medical schools at the point of graduation and four months after graduation, focus groups with junior doctors, interviews with consultants who supervise junior doctors, questionnaires to graduates and giving prescribing tests to graduates. Research was also carried out into prescribing competencies and into the impact of the 1993 *Tomorrow's Doctors*. The results also highlighted concerns which the GMC were already aware of that there have been concerns in recent years about the scientific knowledge base of graduates. This led some doctors and some senior consultants to argue that the recommendations of the 1993 *Tomorrow's Doctors* had gone too far (Williams and Lau, 2004).

A report called 'Junior doctors in the NHS: Preparing medical students for employment and postgraduate training' was also published by Skills for Health as part of the consultation on the draft *Tomorrow's Doctors* 2009. This involved 230 semi-structured interviews with a range of NHS staff across the UK. It must be stressed that many interviewees felt junior doctors were excellent and overall standards were improving. However, as with the research commissioned by the GMC, it did highlight some areas of concern including science knowledge, professionalism, prescribing knowledge of junior doctors and knowledge about NHS guidelines.

The 2009 version of *Tomorrow's Doctors* has taken these specific concerns into account, updating and reformulating the recommendations while retaining the philosophies espoused in the original document. All medical schools and a wide range of stakeholders with an interest in undergraduate medical education had the opportunity to submit their views either by face-to-face meetings or via written proposals on a number of draft versions.

What's the evidence?

The evidence from the research concluded that:

- Graduates look forward to being a doctor, but the transition from student to doctor was experienced as a 'step up' in responsibility and involved a steep learning curve.
- Communication is a strong area at graduation but F1s were under-prepared for complex communication tasks including breaking bad news, distressed or angry patients and dealing with challenging colleagues.
- Clinical skills are well practised as undergraduates but not in contexts which sufficiently mimic the real clinical environment involving multiple demands on time, the need to prioritise and the responsibility of dealing with acute cases.
- Knowledge of some clinical areas, such as legal and ethical issues and the operation of the NHS, was lacking at the start of the F1 year. It did grow during this year, but only regarding their local NHS environment.
- Prescribing is a significant area of under-preparedness. Undergraduate teaching does not prepare new graduates for prescribing as a skilled task involving applied clinical pharmacology. There is a perceived lack of focus on common prescribing tasks and the complexities of interactions and pharmacokinetics.

The following recommendations were made:

- Medical schools should ensure that undergraduate clinical placements have more structure and consistency with experiential learning across a range of specialties.

- Medical students should be given a greater role on medical teams, with due regard to patient safety. Clinical placements should move the student systematically to a more central role before they take on the responsibilities of an F1.
- Fuller, more prescriptive guidelines on the structure and content of shadowing should be established and it should be ensured that F1s have shadowed their job which does not include induction.
- The perceived weakness in prescribing should be addressed by supporting the development of ward-based teaching of prescribing as a skilled procedure which is subject to the time pressures and contingencies of all clinical skills.

Illing, J, Peile, E and Morrison, J and others (2008) *How Prepared Are Medical Graduates to Begin Practice? A Comparison of Three Diverse Medical Schools*. Final Report for the GMC Education Committee. London: GMC.

Skills for Health (2009) *Junior Doctors in the NHS: Preparing Medical Students for Employment and Postgraduate Training*. www.skillsforhealth.org.uk/-/media/Resource-Library/PDF/Tomorrows-Doctors-2009.ashx (accessed 22 October 2010).

ACTIVITY 2.2

Read through both the 1993 and 2009 *Tomorrow's Doctors*. What strikes you about the similarities and differences? Your medical school or library should have copies and they are both available on the internet (www.gmc-uk.org/education/undergraduate/historic_policy.asp and www.gmc-uk.org/education/undergraduate/tomorrows_doctors_2009.asp). Look at both the content and the language and note the different styles.

Summary of the content of *Tomorrow's Doctors* (2009)

The aim of the document is for medical schools to educate students so they can work as competent first-year graduates (see Chapter 11 for details on the current structure of postgraduate training in the UK). The foreword to the document states specifically that the GMC has responded to concerns about scientific education and clinical skills and providing leadership. There is also an emphasis on putting patients first that 'medicine involves personal interaction with people as well as the application of science and technical skills'. It stresses that doctors need to work towards continuous improvement both in their own practice and the environment in which they work.

The introduction highlights again what the GMC is responsible for regarding regulating medical education, specifically including promoting the high standards of medical education and ensuring that universities maintain high standards of teaching. It also stresses, however, the responsibilities for medical schools, the NHS doctors and students. For medical schools these include ensuring that only students who meet the required standards of *Tomorrow's Doctors* and EU directives can graduate. For the NHS these include supporting medical schools in complying with *Tomorrow's Doctors*, releasing doctors and other staff to train to be teachers and making facilities available to support the clinical side of the curriculum. Doctors should follow the principles of professional practice laid out in *Good Medical Practice* and supervise students, ensuring patient safety. Finally, the expectations on the students include being responsible for their own learning, achieving all outcomes in *Tomorrow's Doctors*, whatever their personal or religious beliefs, ensuring patient safety and keeping professional values and that they are fit to practise. The document then goes on to summarise its outcomes for graduates and standards for the delivery of teaching, learning and assessment. The following paragraphs will very briefly summarise these.

The first outcome for graduates is 'the doctor as a scholar and a scientist' and states the graduates should be able to apply medical practice, biomedical scientific principles and knowledge of a range of sciences, including anatomy, pharmacology, pathology and physiology and should have scientific understanding of disease processes, both prevention and management, and have knowledge of the psychological effects of disease. The second outcome is in the domain of 'doctor as practitioner' and concerns the skills the graduate will need to carry out a consultation with patients, including history and examination skills, diagnosing, communicating, prescribing and undertaking practical procedures. Outcome three outlines the 'doctor as a professional' including their duties to keep up to date with latest GMC guidelines, protect patients, reflect and show care and consideration to patients and colleagues. Appendix 1 of the document lists the practical procedures students should learn as an undergraduate, ranging from measuring body temperature and pulse rate to skin suturing and venepuncture.

There are nine domains under the heading 'Standards for the delivery of teaching, learning and assessment' as summarised briefly in Table 2.1. These show that the GMC is not just concerned with skills outcomes, but also with the welfare of students and equality for students as well.

Table 2.1 Summary of the standards for the delivery of teaching

Domain 1 Patient safety	Highlights patient safety and how students and their supervisors should be aware of this in all undergraduate consultations. If there is anything a student doesn't understand such as the practical procedures they should ask an older student, qualified doctor or clinical skills tutor
Domain 2 Quality assurance, review and evaluation	*Tomorrow's Doctors* throughout illustrates how these outcomes and domains can be met and assessed
Domain 3 Equality, diversity and opportunity	Undergraduate medical education must be fair and based on principles of equality

Domain 4 Student selection	Medical schools will publish their admissions criteria and student selection will be 'open, objective and fair'
Domain 5 Design, delivery of the curriculum including assessment	Stresses that medical curricula must be designed and assessed so graduates can demonstrate outcomes in *Tomorrow's Doctors*
Domain 6 Support and development of students, teachers and the local faculty	Shows how students should be supported throughout their time as undergraduates including when they are not progressing well and what pastoral system should be in place to all students, and also what in return is expected of students who after all are training to be doctors
Domain 7 Management of teaching, learning and assessment	Says that medical schools should have a management plan to show who is responsible for delivering all aspects of the curriculum including planning and evaluation
Domain 8 Educational resources and capacity	Stresses that students must have access to all the learning resources they need including libraries, computers, lecture theatres and seminar rooms
Domain 9 Outcomes	Again, the GMC states that medical schools must provide a programme which meets the outcomes in *Tomorrow's Doctors* and finally students must have access to analysis of assessments and examinations at medical school

---

ACTIVITY 2.3

What do you think are the most important aspects of the latest *Tomorrow's Doctors* in preparing you to work as a junior doctor in the future?

Chapter summary

The GMC has established clear guidelines for UK medical schools to follow. The guidelines in *Tomorrow's Doctors* are designed to help prepare graduates to work and train as junior doctors.

GOING FURTHER

- Brennan, N, Corrigan, O and Allard, J (2010) The transition from medical student: today's experiences of *Tomorrow's Doctors*. *Medical Education*, 44: 449–458.
  The research covered in this paper took place about the same time as the two reports below were being published and shows similar conclusions.

- Illing, J, Peile, E and Morrison, J (2008) *How Prepared Are Medical Graduates to Begin Practice? A Comparison of Three Diverse Medical Schools*. Final Report for the GMC Education Committee. London: GMC.
  This report informed the content of Tomorrow's Doctors *(2009).*

- Skills for Health (2009) *Junior Doctors in the NHS: Preparing Medical Students for Employment and Postgraduate Training*. www.skillsforhealth.org.uk/~/media/Resource-Library/PDF/Tomorrows-Doctors-2009.ashx (accessed 22 October 2010).
  This report also informed the content of Tomorrow's Doctors *(2009).*

- Williams, G and Lau, A (2004) Reform of undergraduate medical teaching in the United Kingdom: a triumph of evangelism over common sense. *British Medical Journal*, 329: 92.
  This article highlights some of the concerns that some clinicians had about the original Tomorrow's Doctors.

- Also link to the GMC website Undergraduate Education section as there are lots of resources there which describe the content and rationale of medical education: www.gmc-uk.org/education/undergraduate.asp

chapter 3

Professionalism

Helen O'Sullivan

Achieving your medical degree

This chapter will help you to begin to meet the following requirements of *Tomorrow's Doctors* (GMC, 2009a):

Outcomes 3 – The doctor as a professional

Paragraphs 20–23.

Chapter overview

In this chapter we will examine the concept of medical professionalism. Developing professionalism is seen as increasingly important in medical schools. We will start by understanding why it is important for doctors and medical students to be professional and what 'being professional' means in practice. You will get the opportunity to analyse your own curriculum for learning opportunities for professionalism and prepare for the way that your medical school will assess professionalism. Finally, a case study will help you to appreciate the impact that lack of professional behaviour can have on future career aspirations.

After reading this chapter you will be able to:

- understand why it is important for doctors and medical students to display professional attitudes and behaviour;
- define professionalism in general terms and understand the definition that is used in your medical school;
- understand fitness to practise, both from the point of view of the General Medical Council (GMC) and your own medical school;
- identify learning opportunities to develop professionalism, recognise the impact of the 'hidden curriculum' and be able to reflect on your learning experiences;
- appreciate that a commitment to personal development and high professional standards is a fundamental part of your future career for the rest of your career.

Why is it important for doctors to be professional?

The public come into contact with doctors in a range of different contexts; mostly in hospitals and general practice but also in the media, at the school gate and in the supermarket. We know that they come into contact with doctors at some of the most difficult points in their lives; for example at the beginning of a long and difficult illness, when they are frightened or in pain or as a dearly loved relative is reaching the end of their life. At these points, the patient wants to be able to trust their doctor with decisions that will have a major impact on their lives. It is crucial that a doctor's attitudes and behaviour supports and develops that trust. When the public is asked what makes a good doctor they often say communication, empathy and care. The public takes it for granted that doctors have good medical knowledge and it is other skills, such as 'being a professional' that enable a patient to trust the individual.

What's the evidence?

The Picker Institute is an organisation that looks at how patients' views can be better used in planning health care. This report: www.pickereurope.org/Filestore/ PIE_reports/project_reports/Trends_2007_final.pdf gives a summary of what patients think about professionalism and doctors. The most common criticism of doctors is that the way that they communicate with patients could be improved.

ACTIVITY 3.1

As has been discussed in Chapters 1 and 2, one of the roles of the GMC is to regulate the behaviour of doctors registered with it. The GMC issues guidance on the 'Duties of a doctor' which sets out these standards. Go on to the GMC webpage and find the statement on the 'Duties of a doctor'. See www.gmc-uk.org/guidance/ good_medical_practice/duties_of_a_doctor.asp

For each sentence of the statement, think whether the duty relates to (a) scientific knowledge, (b) technical skills or (c) personal or professional values and attributes. What is the balance between the types of duties required?

This quotation, taken from the preface of *Tomorrow's Doctors* 2009, shows that the GMC expects medical schools to take teaching and assessing professionalism at least as importantly as scientific knowledge and technical skills:

Medical schools equip medical students with the scientific background and technical skills they need for practice. But, just as importantly, they must enable new graduates to both understand and commit to high personal and professional values. Medicine involves personal interaction with people, as well as the application of science and technical skills.

(GMC, 2009a, page 4)

Therefore, the GMC wants you to behave like medical professionals even while you are students.

In the rest of this chapter we will look some definitions of medical professionalism and how you can use the learning opportunities at medical school to ensure that you graduate as a developing professional who will be respected by your patients and peers.

What is medical professionalism and why has it come to prominence?

Many writers and commentators have suggested that the increased interest in medical professionalism has been sparked by some major medical scandals that have taken place in the last few years such as the conviction of Dr Harold Shipman for mass murder, the organ retention scandal in Alder Hey Children's Hospital and the Bristol Royal Infirmary children's heart surgery scandal. Although these may have contributed to a media image of doctors, on the whole, the public still trust doctors more than any other professional group (Royal College of Physicians, 2009).

A more likely explanation for the increasing interest in professionalism is that there have been significant changes in society over the last 20 years and the informal 'societal' contract between doctors and patients has undergone remarkable changes. In the early years of the National Health Service (NHS) patients were passive and enormously grateful to receive the 'wisdom', knowledge and care that a doctor bestowed upon them. They believed that 'doctor knows best' and there was great deference to doctors by both patients and other colleagues in the health service team. Now there is much less automatic respect for authority, an increased informality in public life and the deference that was once shown to doctors seems out of place and old-fashioned.

With the growth of information that is available online, there is also a democratisation of knowledge, and patients are likely to turn up for a consultation being reasonably well informed about their condition and questioning decisions about treatment. Doctors are much more likely to see themselves as part of a health care team and when appropriate will defer to a leader from another health care professional. The recent White Paper on NHS reform includes the phrase 'We want the principle of "shared decision-making" to become the norm: no decision about me without me' indicating that the era of doctors making decisions for patients in what they believe are their best interests is over (NHS, 2010).

Many medical educators have attempted to reflect these changes by defining medical professionalism. These are often lists of attributes or values and there is a good deal of common ground between these definitions. One of the most enduring definitions has been produced by the Royal College of Physicians as an outcome from a working group on medical professionalism. The report, *Doctors in Society*, concludes that medical professionalism 'signifies a set of values, behaviours, and relationships that underpins the trust the public has in doctors' (RCP, 2005, p xi).

In addition, David Stern (a medical educator working in the USA) has defined professionalism graphically as shown in Figure 3.1.

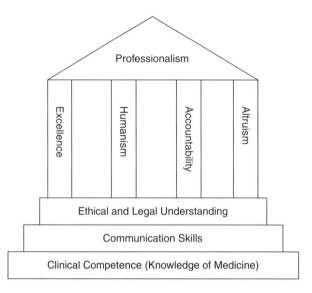

Figure 3.1 A graphical representation of professionalism in medicine © David Stern (2006).

ACTIVITY 3.2

Which of these definitions is the most useful to you? Find out if your medical school has a specific definition of professionalism and compare it with the definitions offered by David Stern and the Royal College of Physicians presented here. Note the similarities and differences between them.

How do medical students develop professionalism?

ACTIVITY 3.3

The following is a quotation from a recent report about what students think about professionalism: 'If I know my consultant has a ward round on a Tuesday and a Friday I dress sharp on a Tuesday and a Friday for that. . . . And then, as soon as the consultant turns round, I loosen my tie or put down my hair' (Levenson *et al.*, 2010). What would the consultant think about the students' professional attitude? How would this come across to patients and other students?

What's the evidence?

In a project that was a partnership between the Royal College of Physicians, The King's Fund, the University of Liverpool, the NHS Institute for Innovation and Improvement, the Student BMJ and the GMC, a series of roadshow events were put on in medical schools across the UK. The views of students about professionalism were listened to and a set of particular questions were posed to groups of students (Levenson et al., 2010). Some of the key issues that came up in this report are that students would like to have more leadership development during their degree and that there is a need to engage students more with the regulatory frameworks set out by the GMC.

In very broad terms, your whole time at medical school and everything that you do during your studies contributes to development of professionalism and ultimately the sort of doctor you will become. All of the time you are in a workplace, you are observing colleagues who will influence your behaviour either by providing a good role model (someone who you aspire to be like) or a bad role model (someone who makes you question their behaviour and whether you would like to be like them). This interaction with role models is often called the 'hidden curriculum' (Hafferty, 1998) because how you develop professionally can be influenced in ways that are unacknowledged. Sometimes the 'hidden curriculum' can have an adverse effect on your development.

ACTIVITY 3.4

In a multiprofessional learning group in medical school two third-year medical students work on a project with two nurse students, a student occupational therapist and a dental student. They receive guidance on how to work as part of a team, how to co-operate with other health care providers and when to take on leadership and when to display followership.

Later that week, the medical students are on a surgical rotation with a renowned surgeon who is responsible for signing off their placement. The surgeon is rude to a theatre nurse, over-rules the view of a registrar and shouts at the medical students because neither of them can recall a particular fact about anatomy.

Which experience is likely to have the most lasting impact on the students' behaviour?

Most successful doctors, however, talk about very positive role models who played a significant role in their development at medical school or as a junior doctor. These colleagues inspired their juniors with the exemplary behaviour and helped them to develop into the excellent professionals that they have become.

Learning opportunities in professionalism

All medical schools must provide opportunities to enable students to develop as professionals, and it is useful to have a look at your own medical school and see what specific activities there are. Some curricula has very explicit strands in the curriculum that pertain to professionalism with others choosing to make professionalism more implicit and integrated. Most schools are somewhere between this. All schools will have explicit activities in communication and ethics and law which are important parts of professionalism, but may not be labelled professionalism.

Although medical students may enjoy the same social and recreational activities as other students, especially in the first few years where you might be in halls of residence with other students, it is important to recognise that, as students on a professional programme, you will be held to higher standards of behaviour than other students. Perhaps the most immediate impact of unprofessional behaviour will fall on your peers. If you turn up late to sessions, skip lectures and ask to borrow notes and attend practical classes with a hangover you will soon become unpopular with your peers. Other students are extremely perceptive at recognising unprofessional behaviour (see Chapter 9 on peer feedback for further discussion of this).

Don't forget that patients have the right to decline to be seen by medical students and if you do not conduct yourself in a professional manner in a clinical setting you may be risking valuable learning opportunities if the patient refuses to let you be involved in their treatment. These standards are directly linked to the standards that you will be held to when you are a doctor. Also, you may need a reference from clinicians who teach you on clinical placements and clinicians are unlikely to give references to students they deem to have acted in an unprofessional manner. Chapter 10 on clinical placements discusses professional behaviour on clinical attachments. All medical schools publish what is known as fitness to practise (FTP) guidance and procedures.

It is really important that you understand the sort of behaviour that could have an impact on your future career; remember, you will need a reference to support your foundation programme application!

ACTIVITY 3.5

Have a detailed look at your medical school's curriculum and guidance about professionalism. Are there specific sessions, lectures or activities on professionalism? Note down the guidance that your school publishes about professional behaviour and FTP. Go on to the GMC website and find the section entitled 'Medical students: professional values and fitness to practise'. This section outlines the professional behaviour expected of medical students and the sorts of behaviour that will probably result in an FTP hearing. Are medical students held to account differently than, say, history students in your university?

Case study: Making wise choices

Lucy is a third-year medical student and is a member of many student societies and sports teams. She has an excellent academic record and has never had any issues with professionalism or behaviour. She is popular with other students and feels that she gets on really well with the patients that she has had contact with up to now.

Lucy is an avid user of social networking sites and has a mobile phone with a camera that she uses to document her life online. Lucy doesn't really understand the privacy settings on the site but is reasonably sure that only her friends can see what she posts. One Saturday afternoon, Lucy takes a break from studying to update her favourite social networking site page. In the space of an hour Lucy:

- uploads pictures of the recent medical student hockey tour 'end of tour party' showing students who have been drinking heavily engaged in juvenile behaviour wearing sweatshirts clearly identifying the medical school that they are all at;
- accepts a friend request from someone she doesn't know;
- posts a comment on her sister's site in reply to a request for advice about the side-effects of a drug that has been prescribed to Lucy's 5-year-old nephew;
- clicks the 'I like this' response to a mildly homophobic joke sent to her by a fellow medical student;
- tags an acquaintance in a photograph posted by another medical student;
- discusses a rare clinical case with a fellow student in enough detail to risk identifying the patient;
- vents her frustration at being on the receiving end of some sarcastic comments from a senior consultant during that week's clinical attachment;
- joins the jokey public group 'Doctors for Devil Worship' (as it is nearly Halloween).

ACTIVITY 3.6

For each action in the case study above, decide whether Lucy has been or is at risk of being unprofessional. Using these specific actions as examples, what general guidance would you give to fellow medical students about how they use social media?

Professionalism, reflection and insight

One of the key attributes of a successful professional doctor is the ability to reflect on their own learning and behaviour, to have insight into that behaviour and to be able to identify their own strengths and weaknesses. This insight is difficult to achieve as it needs to strike a balance between underestimating your abilities and being over confident or cocky. Having appropriate confidence in your abilities means that you will be trusted as a good colleague by your peers and will be less likely to make mistakes that have a negative outcome on patient safety. By recognising your weakness (or 'development needs' as they are often euphemistically called!) with humility but not causing undue personal distress you can work on putting them right. If you make a mistake, accept responsibility for that mistake and learn from it and move on.

It is useful (and often great fun!) to learn more about your personality type, your learning style and how you perform in a team. Your university will have a Careers Department that will probably offer a range of personal development tools such as learning style inventories or Myers Briggs Personality Type Indicator (see also Chapter 11 on careers). If not, there are many online sites that provide these sorts of inventories and offer some analysis

---

ACTIVITY 3.7

Start to keep a personal learning journal for professionalism. This can be in any format (a small notebook, an actual diary or electronically) and should note learning opportunities in any aspect of professionalism. For example, you might see a junior doctor staying well past the end of her shift so that she can explain in person what is happening to the relative of a dying patient. On the other hand, you might witness a senior clinician snapping at a junior colleague because they have made a relatively minor mistake. In each case, write down what it was about the incident that you thought made the behaviour or attitude professional or unprofessional and how you could learn from the experience. It is also useful to note down situations when your own professionalism was tested and your reaction to that.

Assessment of professionalism

Medical schools use a variety of ways to assess students on their professionalism and give them feedback. The most common approaches currently in use are peer assessment, the objective structured clinical examination (OSCE), direct observation of procedural skills (sometimes called DOPS), mini-clinical examinations (often called mini-CEX), critical incidents reports and reflective portfolios. Use of standardised checklists, written comments and comments from formal evaluation sessions completed by a supervisor and/or other staff is frequent. Other methods of assessing of professional behaviour include the writing of short narratives (sometimes called critical incident reports) and self-assessment (see also Chapter 5 on assessment).

Often one method of assessment is used to assess a number of different skills or attributes. A good example of this is the OSCE that is used to assess clinical skills but is often used to assess communication and professionalism at the same time.

It is important to be really clear about the purpose of the assessment. All assessment should contain an element of feedback and if you receive a mark or a comment in a way that you can't learn from it you should tactfully request some further feedback.

Case study: One night out

John has just graduated from medical school with an exemplary academic record and a prize for the best mark in the student selected components of his year group. He has his heart set on a career in one of the most competitive specialties and has been doing additional work experience in that area to boost his career chances. He has decided to apply for a foundation post at the most prestigious hospital in the country in this specialty so that he can further develop links and work in his chosen area. When John was at the start of his second year, he was helping his medical school student society organise a 'freshers'' event that included a pub crawl of high profile bars and pubs in the city centre where he was studying. The pub crawl got out of hand and John, along with some others, was arrested and charged with an offence linked to being drunk. He came forward with the information to his medical school and went through the university's fitness to practise procedure. The university accepted that the behaviour was out of character and allowed John to continue with his studies but an outcome of the process was that a note of the event was to be held on John's student record. John was not offered a training post at his preferred hospital and had to accept a post in a Deanery in a part of the country where he had no family or friends and in a hospital that was not a specialty centre in his preferred career. He was left wondering what part, if any, the incident in his second year had played in the foundation application process.

Striving for personal excellence

I hope that reading this chapter has inspired you to take forward your professional development with pride. As a medical student, you are already used to working very hard and achieving the highest academic standards. In medical school, you have many competing demands on your time and you are now in a cohort of the brightest and most able students in the university system. It can sometimes be hard to maintain the conscientiousness that got you here in the first place, especially if no one is looking and you can 'get away with it'. All doctors and medical students are human and it might be that you have had a row with your partner or you are feeling under the weather and feel that you can't be bothered to be cheerful to the elderly lady in bed 3 who has a reputation for being grumpy and complaining. Remember that the genuine professional (student or doctor) is one who holds themselves to the highest personal standards, even when no one is looking.

Chapter summary

In this chapter you have covered the following aspects of professionalism:

- definitions of professionalism and why it is important for doctors to be professional;

- why medical schools are teaching medical professionalism and how students can develop as professionals;

- the ways in which you can ensure that you make the most of the learning opportunities for professionalism and how professionalism is assessed;

- the role that reflection and insight plays in personal development and the importance of striving for professional excellence.

GOING FURTHER

- Anon. (2010) Physician know thyself. *Lancet*, 376(9743): 743.
  The Student BMJ *and the* Lancet *often have editorials or opinion pieces about professionalism. For example, the article included here discusses the issue of doctors and their religious beliefs and the potential for conflict of interest.*

- Royal College of Physicians (2005) *Doctors in Society: Medical Professionalism in a Changing World.* London: RCP.
  The original report of the working group of the Royal College of Physicians is a particularly interesting review of what doctors think about medical professionalism.

chapter 4

Medical Leadership

Helen O'Sullivan

Achieving your medical degree

This chapter will help you to begin to meet the following requirements of *Tomorrow's Doctors* (GMC, 2009a):

Outcomes 3 – The doctor as a professional

Paragraphs 21–23 and in particular paragraph 22(d): 'Demonstrate ability to build team capacity and positive working relationships and undertake various team roles including leadership and the ability to accept leadership by others.'

Paragraph 7 (Outcomes for graduates) makes it clear that leadership is a central part of what it takes to be a medical graduate:

'In accordance with Good Medical Practice, graduates will make the care of patients their first concern, applying their knowledge and skills in a competent and ethical manner and using their ability to provide leadership and to analyse complex and uncertain situations.' (GMC, 2009a)

Chapter overview

In this chapter we will examine the concept of medical leadership. By looking at the importance of medical leadership you will begin to appreciate how to develop the skills of leadership (and management) that you will need in your future career as a doctor. A key document, the *Medical Leadership Competency Framework* is introduced and specific examples of how the Framework could be used are given. Finally, the concept of followership is discussed and highlighted with a case study.

After reading this chapter you will be able to:

- understand why it is important for doctors and medical students to offer leadership to patients, their families and other colleagues;
- define medical leadership;
- understand that there are differences between leadership and management but realise that there are significant overlaps;
- identify the particular importance of followership in being a successful doctor;
- appreciate that team working and multiprofessional working are a crucial aspect of professional life.

Why do doctors need leadership training?

It is not enough for a clinician to act as a practitioner in their own discipline. They must act as partners to their colleagues, accepting shared accountability for the service provided to their patients. They are also expected to offer leadership and to work with others to change systems when it is necessary for the benefit of patients.

This quotation from *Tomorrow's Doctors* (GMC, 2009a) explains why leadership development is now an important part of undergraduate curricula. In the past, doctors were seen as the automatic leaders in any health care situation and other health care professionals, as well as patients and their families, showed an automatic deference to authority figures. Nowadays, however, as has already been highlighted in Chapters 1, 2 and 3, things are more complicated! Changes in society mean that automatic deference to perceived authority figures is rarer and health care teams include many different specialties.

As a doctor, you will often be expected to offer leadership to patients and their families, to members of the various health care teams, to junior doctors and students and, sometimes, to other doctors. In fact as a senior GP or consultant you may well in effect be a 'line manager' to junior doctors. Also, some doctors choose to give up some or all of their clinical work and become senior managers in hospitals or senior civil servants in the Department of Health or work in bodies such as the British Medical Association or GMC. Just as importantly, sometimes you will be expected to accept leadership from others. This concept is known as 'followership' and will be discussed later in the chapter. Leadership is fundamentally about having a vision and then motivating people to work with you towards that vision. Communicating the vision, building trust, empowering people and working in teams are also important. It should be clear to you that a lot of the skills required to be a good leader are complementary to those of being a good doctor.

ACTIVITY 4.1

Think back to any work experience in a health care setting that you had before coming to medical school or to any placements that you have been on so far. Think about a doctor who you have really admired. Obviously they will have had good clinical skills, but think about the personal qualities that they had. How did they communicate with colleagues and patients? Were they calm under pressure? How did they prioritise and organise their time? Chances are you have just described the qualities of a good medical leader!

Many of the qualities of a good leader overlap with professionalism (see Chapter 3 as well for more details on professionalism) and in many medical schools, leadership, team working and teaching as seen as part of the broader professionalism agenda. Your values as a leader will be strongly influenced by your values as a professional and it would be useful to be clear about these values before you consider your development as a leader.

What's the evidence?

A recent review article by Warren and Parnell (2011) 'Medical leadership: why it's important, what is required, and how we develop it' outlines the evidence behind a range of reasons why it is important to develop leadership skills in junior doctors and outlines some of the ways that leadership is being assessed in postgraduate training.

Management and leadership – do all doctors need to be managers and leaders?

ACTIVITY 4.2

Think of someone that you consider to be an inspirational leader. It doesn't have to be from the medical world, it could be a politician, a business leader, a sporting, cultural or community leader. Write down five words that describe what makes them special as a leader. Next write down five words that come to mind when you think of the word 'manager'. What are the differences between the two?

There is often some confusion about what constitutes a leader or manager in the medical context. In the recent report entitled *The 21st Century Doctor: Understanding the Doctors of Tomorrow*, a medical student commented:

Obviously, leadership is an important part of management but every doctor is a leader . . . even the junior doctors are leaders in respect to the medical students, a fourth year is a leader in respect to a third year, they're all teachers but managers are leaders in an organisational sense where as all doctors are leaders.

(Levenson *et al.*, 2010, page 36)

Although many writers have attempted to distinguish between leadership and management, this quotation draws a clear and relevant distinction for medical students and junior doctors.

In the last few years there has been a move towards non-doctors taking more responsibility for managing clinical services. In his influential report about the future of the health service, however, Lord Darzi comments: 'Making change actually happen takes leadership. It is central to our expectations of the healthcare professions of tomorrow' (Darzi, 2008). At the time of writing, the NHS is undergoing another structural reorganisation and it is probably safe to assume that change and the management of change will be a key feature of your career. By developing leadership and management skills and competencies while you are a medical student and a junior doctor, you will be well placed to take a role in deciding the direction and clinical priorities for the health service that you will be working in.

Engaging the medical community with medical leadership

What's the evidence?

After some difficulties with the implementation of the Modernising Medical Careers (MMC) reforms (see Chapter 11), Sir John Tooke (who was then Dean of the Peninsula Medical School) was asked by the government to lead an independent enquiry into how MMC had been implemented. The resultant report (known colloquially as the Tooke Report) contains the following key paragraph that has had a significant impact on the way that leadership and management training are viewed in medical education:

The doctor's frequent role as head of the healthcare team and commander of considerable clinical resource requires that greater attention is paid to management and leadership skills regardless of specialism. An acknowledgement of the leadership role of medicine is increasingly evident. Role acknowledgement and aspiration to enhanced roles be they in subspecialty practice, management and leadership, education or research are likely to facilitate greater clinical engagement.

(Tooke, 2008)

Medical Leadership Competency Framework

In response to the need for doctors to become more actively involved in the review, planning, delivery and transformation of health services the Academy of Medical Royal Colleges and the NHS Institute for Innovation and Improvement in conjunction with a wide range of stakeholders set up a UK-wide project called 'Enhancing Engagement in Medical Leadership'. One of the outcomes of this project was the *Medical Leadership Competency Framework*. This Framework describes the skills and competencies that medical students and doctors need in order to contribute to running successful services. The Framework has five domains: Demonstrating personal qualities, Working with others, Managing services, Improving services and Setting direction. The Framework rightly recognises that not all of these will be as important to medical students so it has a separate section for undergraduate medical education.

Opportunities to develop leadership as an undergraduate

Many medical schools will not have classes or sessions explicitly labelled 'leadership' but there are lots of opportunities to practise and demonstrate leadership skills as an

---

ACTIVITY 4.3

Find the *Medical Leadership Competency Framework* on line (www.institute. nhs.uk/assessment_tool/general/medical_leadership_competency_framework_- _homepage.html). For each of the five domains, look at some of the competencies that are specifically suggested for undergraduates. For each of the domains, write down one competency that you feel you can already demonstrate.

---

undergraduate. Some of these direct leadership activities can be taking leadership of your problem-based learning (PBL) group or other small group classes (volunteering to present to your fellow students) as well as standing for office in your local student medical society. You can also volunteer to assist junior students as you progress through medical school and become more experienced. The rest of this section will discuss some of the ways that you might encounter leadership training during your curriculum relating to the five domains in the *Medical Leadership Competence Framework*.

Demonstrating personal qualities

An important part of developing as a leader is having a clear understanding of your personal qualities and where your strengths and weaknesses lie. Many medical schools make use of a variety of personality and other types of inventories to help you explore these aspects. Some of the most useful types of inventories are those that give you an insight into your learning style or your group working style. The Myers Briggs Personality Type Indicator (discussed in more detail in Chapter 11) is a particularly useful way of looking at your personality and understanding the working types of your colleagues. If your medical school does not offer this sort of testing, you may be able to get it from your University Careers Service or skills development unit. You should reflect on the outcome and think about how the results explain the way that you work or react to certain situations and can help you develop.

You can practise some of the personal qualities that are important in leadership by volunteering to lead seminars or other small groups, or take part in objective structured clinical examinations (OSCEs). Many medical schools now offer the opportunity to undertake some form of appraisal, some with what is known as 360-degree feedback. This type of appraisal can involve students getting feedback on their personal qualities and professional values from a variety of sources (the 360 refers to 360°, the internal angle of a circle, and suggests that you, the student, are at the centre of the circle and that you are getting feedback from all points of that circle around you). This should be viewed as an opportunity to set goals in your personal development planning and can offer insights into your personal qualities that are appreciated by your colleagues, as well as, occasionally, areas that you might need to work on!

Working with others

Your time in medical school is a rich environment for practising team working skills and demonstrating that you can work well with others. All curricula provide some form of small group teaching which, as highlighted above, is ideal for practising leading a group. In addition, you will be expected to work co-operatively with other students in clinical placements and when studying practical skills such as clinical skills or communication skills classes. In addition, many schools have opportunities to work with other health care students as part of multidisciplinary team working. The multidisciplinary team can include nurses, physiotherapists, occupational therapists and social workers, for example. This might range from being taught communication skills or clinical skills with other students to undertaking entire group tasks as part of a multidisciplinary student team. Also, many primary care centres have therapists and community nurses based in them as well as GPs.

ACTIVITY 4.4

During your next clinical placement, investigate the range of job title and specialties that make up the 'health care team'. Don't forget workers from other sectors such as social workers. Ask a manager to look at your list to see if you have missed anyone out. Use the internet to do a quick review of the scope of each role that you have on your list and reflect how you might be called to work with them when you are a doctor.

One of the most effective ways of improving your team working is to get feedback from the people who know you best – your fellow medical students! Peer feedback is becoming increasingly used in medical curricula to help you develop ways of improving the way you relate to your colleagues. Giving feedback and receiving it are important skills that need to be developed; they don't necessarily come easily. In fact, receiving feedback can be difficult and it is important not to take it personally. In the same way, it can be really hard to give negative feedback to a colleague who has come to be a friend. Both of these can become easier with some training and development (Garner et al., 2010) and will be discussed in more detail in Chapter 9.

There are also opportunities to demonstrate skills of working with and leading others in activities outside the formal curriculum. Sport, music, community and charity work as well as trips abroad during electives or vacations can offer valuable experiences. Medical students are extremely good at working with other year groups! This work is particular valuable for developing team work, followership and leadership skills. In the first few years use more senior students as a resource for feedback and to practise followership and team work. A soon as you get the opportunity, look for ways to work with more junior years practising teaching skills and leadership skills.

Managing services

As well as possibly having lectures or small group classes on the structure and function of the main health care providers, you will be spending a large proportion of your time as a student in the health care settings that you will be eventually working in. Take advantage of opportunities to talk to patients and their families about their experience of health care, how the different aspects of primary and secondary care work together and reflect on their frustrations and positive experiences. There may be opportunities to shadow a health care manager and start to understand the complexities of managing services. In preparation for leading others, there may also be formal or informal opportunities to design and deliver educational activities for peers, junior students or even schoolchildren who are attending open days at your medical school.

Improving services

During the later years of your course there will be opportunities to take part in formal audits or other projects to explore improving services. These usually take the form of special projects, electives or student selected components (see Chapter 8). These are really useful ways of starting to understand some of the issues around improving services, especially economic considerations. One of the crucial skills in improving services is being able to think analytically and to be constantly curious about how things could be done better.

Setting direction

This is perhaps the most difficult aspect of the *Medical Leadership Competency Framework* to demonstrate as a medical student. Setting the direction is about contributing to the strategic direction of the organisation and providing evidence-based challenges to systems and processes in order to identify opportunities for service improvement. As well as the opportunity to demonstrate these skills you will also have lots of opportunity to practise the component parts such as evaluating impact, making decisions and applying knowledge and evidence.

ACTIVITY 4.5

Look at the curriculum for your current year in your medical school. Are there any specific activities or outcomes that mention leadership? See if you can map your curriculum onto the *Medical Leadership Competency Framework*. It is unlikely that the curriculum will mention specific activities or outcomes for each competency but you will be able to map other activities (such as small group work). Once you have finished with your curriculum mapping, think about the activities that you do outside of studying. Do any of these activities help you to demonstrate leadership competencies?

Followership

Different ways of approaching the organisation of health care rely on different approaches to leadership and team working. A collaborative approach, where there is more shared decision making and working across interdisciplinary boundaries, requires doctors to understand how to work as part of a team and to accept the leadership of others. As a junior doctor you may work with senior specialist nurses who have been working in that specialty for 30 years or more. Also, you may need to follow the advice and guidance of occupational therapists when deciding if one of your patients can be discharged from hospital. All leaders are followers because not only do they have to follow their own leader but they need to understand and take a lead from their own teams.

A good leader should actively seek out difficult opinions and views from their teams so that the decisions they make are fully informed and have the best chance of leading to a successful outcome. Sometimes, however, a leader may make a decision based on incomplete information or a lack of understanding of the implications of their actions. In these cases, someone showing really good followership would have the courage to challenge the leader in a tactful and diplomatic manner. This is an example of active fellowship. Telling a leader something that they may not want to hear is very difficult but it could be the difference between a successful and unsuccessful patient outcome.

As you move through your career, you will observe a gradual shift in the balance between leadership and followership. In the early years of your medical school programme you will be mostly demonstrating followership with some limited opportunities for developing leadership. As you become a senior student and a junior doctor, the balance will shift and there will be opportunities for informal leadership of medical students. As you become a consultant or GP the balance will shift again, with you having responsibility for training junior doctors. However, at each end of the spectrum, both elements will remain as essential components of your professional identity.

What's the evidence?

Barrow et al. (2010) have investigated the nature of leadership and followership in junior doctors and junior nurses and looked at the effect of professional identities and traditional notions of team working and leadership and the ability to accept leadership (i.e. followership) from others. The paper provides some interesting findings about the source of power in multiprofessional teams and makes recommendations for people responsible for nurse and doctor education.

ACTIVITY 4.6

In the research reported in the paper by Barrow *et al.* (2010) the following results were obtained: '70% of nurses thought nurses should make decisions on behalf of an interprofessional team, but 80% of doctors disagreed' (page 7). What issues does this result highlight? Can you think of any ways in which these opposite views could be addressed?

Case study: Asking for help

A woman was brought into a busy obstetrics and gynaecology department in the middle of the night in advanced stages of labour. The midwife examined the woman and was concerned that the unborn baby was showing signs of distress. She called in the junior doctor who was on duty to take a look. He was also concerned and decided to phone the senior consultant who was on call. The senior consultant was very irritated to be called in the night for what she thought was a trivial matter and told the junior to go back and redo all of the tests and only call back if things were critical. After 4 hours, the labour had slowed down but the baby's vital signs were still causing concern. Just before dawn the junior doctor reluctantly called the senior again to report his concerns but because she had been angry before, he played down the seriousness of the baby's condition. When the consultant asked him for his opinion he said that he thought things were probably going OK. The senior said that she was on her way into work and would pop in a soon as she was on the ward and suggested that a drug to speed up labour could be administered if the junior thought it was needed. On returning to the mother, the junior discovered that the baby was now in severe distress and he decided to administer the drug suggested by the senior. The midwife knew that this drug was inappropriate for that stage of labour but thought that she would keep quiet so as not to make the situation anymore stressful for the doctor and patient. When the senior doctor came on duty an hour later, she decided that things were critical and that an emergency caesarean section was needed. Although the baby survived the delivery, the junior doctor was left very shaken by the incident and vowed to learn the valuable lessons of being a good leader and follower.

Chapter summary

This chapter has explained what leadership and followership is within medicine and medical education, including:

- the importance of developing leadership and followership skills as an undergraduate and their relevance for when you work as a doctor;

- how your leadership role will change and evolve through your undergraduate and postgraduate career;

- whatever leadership role a doctor takes they still have to work as part of the team.

GOING FURTHER

- Swanwick, T and McKimm, J (2010) *ABC of Clinical Leadership* (ABC Series). London: Wiley Blackwell.
  This book gives a step-by-step guide to becoming a clinical leader.

chapter 5

Assessment in Medical Education

Ray Fewtrell

Achieving your medical degree

This chapter will help you to begin to meet the following requirements of *Tomorrow's Doctors* (GMC, 2009a):

Domain 5 – Design and delivery of the curriculum, including assessment

Standard 81: The curriculum must be designed, delivered and assessed to ensure that graduates demonstrate all the 'outcomes for graduates' specified in *Tomorrow's Doctors.*

Chapter overview

This chapter will outline the different types and forms of assessment used within medical schools, including knowledge-based, practical, formative, summative and continuous assessment. It will look at the different ways of assessing the components of modern medical curricula and the educational theory behind them. Examination techniques that students can use to assist in their revision and exam taking will be explored. It will also explain how the feedback provided by formative assessment can be utilised by students to improve their future performance. This chapter will include a brief discussion of the methods used in setting pass marks for assessments and describe techniques for being successful in assessments.

After reading this chapter you will be able to:

- understand why assessment is necessary in undergraduate medical curricula;
- gain knowledge of the different forms of assessment;
- understand how to use any provided feedback and how different revision, preparation and examination techniques can aid in your success in assessments;
- understand the process of how the pass marks are set for assessments.

Assessment process

Why is assessment necessary?

It has been well noted in education literature that assessment drives learning (Wass *et al.*, 2001). Therefore, assessment is a vital part of all modern medical curricula; it provides the means for ensuring competence, quality, providing guidance and feedback. The General Medical Council (GMC) outlines the expected standards for assessment in *Tomorrow's Doctors* and ensures that medical schools are meeting these standards during their regular inspections (see Chapters 1 and 2). Different forms of assessment can be used to check that students' knowledge, skills, attitudes and abilities are of the required competencies for a medical degree. Patient safety is an important part of being a doctor and assessment can ensure that medical students are aware of health and safety issues and are competent in their skills and abilities to communicate with and examine patients. Also, final assessments at medical schools ensure students have the required skills and knowledge to work and train as first-year postgraduates.

Assessment continues throughout a practising doctor's career in many forms. Portfolio assessment is used for both appraisal and assessment from foundation year training through to revalidation as a consultant or GP. Doctors applying for specialty training in one of the Royal Colleges (e.g. Royal College of Anaesthetists, Royal College of Surgeons) will be expected to sit 'high stakes' written examinations and practical assessments which are often in similar formats to undergraduate exams.

Feedback provided from assessments can guide a student on their strengths and areas for improvement. This feedback can also provide a means of emphasising important areas of the curriculum for study. The data from assessments can also be used by teachers to gauge the success and effectiveness of certain teaching programmes or methods. The areas of strength and weakness can be gauged from the results of assessment and any areas of weakness in a programme can be revisited to improve student knowledge.

Considerations for assessment

There are many considerations when designing an assessment, and an understanding of these considerations will help students in their approach to the different forms of assessment. Figure 5.1 shows a framework developed to demonstrate different levels of assessment (Miller, 1990). Assessments in medical education are designed to ensure that students will be assessed at all of these levels using different forms of assessment. The lowest level within this pyramid is the assessment of knowledge; this level requires the recall of factual knowledge by students. The second level of the pyramid is assessment that examines whether students know how to apply their knowledge – a good example being assessments that look at how students synthesise information and then describe an appropriate action. The third level of the pyramid is the performance level; these assessments are where students are required to demonstrate their skills at performing particular actions such as a physical examination, procedure or skill. The final level of the pyramid is the action level, where students are assessed on how they respond in real life situations and this form of assessment is mostly carried out within the clinical setting and is done by direct observation of students dealing with patients and colleagues. The pyramid can be considered in two halves: the bottom two sections can be seen as the cognitive levels and the top two sections can been seen as the behavioural levels.

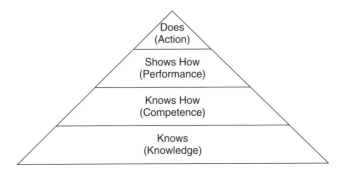

Figure 5.1 Framework for clinical assessment (Miller, 1990). Reproduced with permission.

Several factors need to be considered in assessment, including reliability, validity, feasibility and educational impact. These four elements all need to be balanced to ensure an effective and practical assessment. Reliability measures whether if the same test was performed with the same group of students how similar the results would be; it can be thought of as 'reproducibility'. The validity of an assessment looks at how well the assessment measures the subject. The feasibility of the assessment considers the resources required (e.g. monetary, human, physical and temporal). The impact of the assessment also needs to be considered on both the students' learning and the educational programme.

Assessment methods

There are many different forms of assessment and this section will describe some of the more common types. These different forms of assessment can be divided into written and practical/in-training assessment. Assessments can be referred to as either open or closed book. An open book assessment is where material is provided prior to the assessment and students are permitted to take this material as reference or basis for a particular answer into the assessment. Students are not permitted to take any materials into closed book assessments.

Summative and formative assessment

Summative assessments demonstrate that students have attained a required level of competence or proficiency sufficient to progress to the next stage of training or

course. Summative assessments, referred to as 'high stakes' examinations, usually occur at the end of the year, or include Royal College membership or fellowship examinations. These assessments must be legally defensible for both future
patients, students, the medical school and the GMC. Formative assessments are
designed to monitor student progress and to give students feedback on their
strengths and weaknesses. Formative assessments such as mock exams or progress
tests can give students an idea of the style and format of future summative assessments. Summative and formative assessment may happen at one particular point in
time in the form of an examination or it may occur over a period of time in the form
of continuous assessment.

Written assessments

Written examinations are a form of assessment that occur under strict conditions
with all students sitting the examinations at the same time, typically over a period of
an hour to 3 hours. Written examinations usually test the knowledge level of Miller's
pyramid as it is difficult to assess the competence level using a written examination.
Closed questions are a form of written question where students are provided with
a series of questions with several answers to choose from with one or more being
correct. Multiple choice questions (MCQs) are where a student selects one correct
answer from a series of other distracter items. Extended matching item (EMI) questions are where a series of questions are asked based on a set of answers, some of
which may be used one or multiple times. Each of these EMIs will be on a specific
subject area; the answers within these may also have distracters which are not correct answers for any of the question stems. There also true/false questions which are
closed questions where students must judge whether the statement is correct.

Open assessment questions are questions where the students are not given any
answers to choose from but must answer the questions from their own knowledge.
The responses to the questions may be in the form of a short answer consisting of
one word or a phrase. Longer responses to questions may be in the form of a paragraph or even in the form of an essay. Written examinations may be based directly
on patient cases. Examples of these are key clinical cases or patient management
problems. The written assessment may ask for suggested investigations, examinations and possible diagnoses based on given signs and symptoms. These case-based
examinations use more complex cognitive processes and hence may reach the competence level of Millar's pyramid.

Written assessments can be used for a more continuous form of assessment
than simply examinations. These may be completed over a period of time under
non-examination conditions. These extended assessments may be student selected
components (see Chapter 8), critical incident analysis, reflective exercises, logbooks
and portfolios. All practising clinicians are now required to maintain a portfolio of
practice during their working lives. The portfolios used within undergraduate medical education serve as an introduction for students to the skills required to keep their
postgraduate portfolios. These portfolios provide evidence of students' progress in
their clinical attachments (see Chapter 12).

Practical assessments

Similar to the written assessments, practical assessments can be in the form of an examination or continuous assessment. Practical assessments can assess competence as well as the higher levels of performance and action of Miller's pyramid. Practical examinations may consist of a series of short practical encounters where students move from one station to the next, demonstrating a series of different skills, procedures and examinations in a set amount of time. These station-based examinations may be objective structured clinical examinations (OSCEs), objective structured practical examinations (OSPEs) or communication skills examinations. The stations within these examinations often contain patients, simulated patients or an anatomical/ artificial model for a student to demonstrate a skill, examination or procedure. OSCEs are designed to simulate real patient encounters. For further details on simulation see Chapter 7 and for how communications skills are tested during OSCE examinations see Chapter 6.

Practical-based assessments can also be case based. These require students to take a history and examination from a patient with a particular condition and then review and record the relevant investigations. The students are then required to present and discuss their findings with a clinician. The length and complexity of these cases develops during the clinical years of the programme. These assessments may consist of a few shorter cases or one long case that the students have to discuss. Some universities have created hybrid short case and OSCE (Wass and Van Der Vleuten, 2004) combining the case-based nature of the short cases and the objective structured nature of the OSCE to produce a structured clinical examination that is more consistent for large groups of students.

Practical assessments can occur during clinical attachments. These assessments may be a clerking, examination or practical procedure observed as being of an acceptable standard by a supervising clinician. Some of these assessments have been derived from pre-existing postgraduate in-training assessments. Two common tools are the mini-clinical evaluation exercise (mini-CEX) and direct observation of procedural skills (DOPS). A mini-CEX is a snapshot of a student–patient consultation observed by a clinical supervisor which is designed to assess a student's skills and behaviours to ensure high quality of patient care (Norcini *et al.*, 1995). A DOPS assessment is a structured method of assessing a student performing a practical procedure on a patient. A case-based discussion (CBD) is a common method of assessing a student's clinical cases. In CBDs students will be asked to present one or more clinical cases to a supervising clinician. These CBDs have the strength that they allow the clinician to assess a student's clinical reasoning, presentation skills, history taking and examination skills.

Multi-source assessments have become common in both undergraduate and postgraduate education. Multi-source assessments consist of a series of judgements by peers, supervisors, tutors and patients on a student's behaviour and professionalism demonstrated within a clinical setting. Multi-source assessment can also be referred to as 360-degree assessment or team assessment of behaviour (Whitehouse *et al.*, 2005). Multi-source assessments provide useful feedback regarding actions and competence within clinical placements. This feedback can be included as part of a wider portfolio of evidence of clinical practice.

ACTIVITY 5.1 KINDS OF ASSESSMENT

Find out about the assessments at your medical school; find out the format, length and question style. Which of these assessments do you feel you will have most difficulty with? Think/read about what you can do to relieve this anxiety about this assessment. Talk to peers or more senior students or tutors to find out how they cope with this assessment.

Feedback

Feedback provided by assessments is very important as a learning tool. Providing feedback can help you gauge your strengths and weaknesses in particular areas and help you focus your studies on areas of weakness or development. Feedback can be provided as verbal feedback directly to the student from a tutor or in a written form. Feedback can vary widely in its level of detail from an overall or sectional score to specific feedback on each question or each topic. Feedback should cover what went well and what areas need further work or development.

When receiving verbal feedback you should listen carefully and try to understand the feedback considering the point of view of the person giving the feedback. Attention should be paid to both the positive and the negative comments provided within the feedback. Try not to react to the feedback immediately but reflect and think about all aspects of what was said. Some students find it useful to make notes either during the feedback or immediately after to try to summarise the key points and use these to develop an action plan. The advantage of verbal feedback is that it gives you the opportunity to discuss, clarify and ask further questions to gain the most from the provided feedback.

Similar steps should be conducted when receiving written feedback, including paying attention to positive and negative aspects, making notes on key points and developing an action plan. It can also be useful to categorise the feedback into either topics or specific areas (e.g. grammar, style, knowledge). If you do not understand the feedback it can be helpful to discuss this area with peers and tutors, or try to contact the person delivering the feedback for further explanation.

Case study: Using feedback effectively

Sally, a first-year student sat her short answer formative paper and passed with 68 per cent. A few weeks later she received written feedback from the paper. She was upset and initially annoyed by the feedback as she felt that some of the comments were harsh and overly critical of her answers. She was also annoyed by one particular comment stating that she had only given two out of three required responses to a particular question. She clearly remembered writing three responses to this question. Sally decided she needed an opportunity to discuss this feedback further. She arranged to see her personal tutor to discuss it.

Discussing the feedback with her tutor, the tutor pointed out that although the comments seemed harsh the majority were only minor points within the questions. The tutor reminded Sally that this was a formative exam and the feedback was very useful in preparing her for the summative end-of-year exams. The tutor went on to help Sally organise the comments into specific action points so that she could then target particular areas of study. The tutor then discussed with Sally her answers to the question where the feedback stated that she had only given two out of three responses. When they both looked at Sally's answers to this question it was clear that although she had written three different answers to this question the third answer was just a rewording of the first two answers.

Sally reflected on the conversation with her tutor, the feedback comments and marks she received for her formative exams. Although she still felt that she could have achieved a better mark in her formative exam, she realised there were some areas of improvement she could make ready for her end-of-year exams. A combination of the feedback, discussion with her tutor and good exam preparation techniques led to Sally achieving an 82 per cent pass in the end-of-year exam. Sally felt happy with this result and appreciated the value of the formative exam experience and feedback.

Assessment techniques

This section will cover preparation and assessment techniques, it will give an overview on how you should prepare for assessment and will focus on techniques for getting the best out of written examinations.

Preparation for assessment

It is very important to be prepared for examinations. Not only do you need to know the subject of exam but you should also ensure that you know the style of questions, length of the exam, when and where it occurs and what you are required to take it. Different forms of examinations require students to take particular items with them: for computer-read MCQ exams a pencil is usually required to mark the scheme, for longer written exams some institutions require the answer in a particular colour (e.g. black ink) and for practical exams you may require a stethoscope, a watch and a pocket mask as well as writing equipment. For open book examinations you may be required to take a specific article or paper with you as the basis of an answer.

Revision

People revise in different ways depending on their learning style; many students will have discovered the best methods to revise to be successful for their GCSEs and A-levels. Despite these different learning styles, some techniques are still useful in the preparation for written exams. The use of example questions can be particularly beneficial to ensure that a particular topic is well known. Past papers are a valuable asset as these allow a student to test their knowledge and also become accustomed to the style of the exam. Some tutors provide self-assessment questions; these have the advantage that they have the worked answers so students can ensure that their answers are correct. For some exams neither past papers nor self-assessment questions are available. In this case it can be useful for students to revise in a group. One tactic is for each person in the group to write a couple of questions in the style of the exam and then to ask the rest of the group to complete these questions. Group revision can also be useful as it allows students to discuss topics verbally and can lead to a greater breadth of topics revised.

ACTIVITY 5.2 REVISION

During revision for your next assessment construct five questions of your own relating to areas of the topic that you feel are your own weak points. Revise these topics and then try to answer your own questions in as much detail as possible.

Taking assessments

It is important at the start of any assessment to listen to and read any instructions and guidance carefully. At the start of written exams, ascertain how many questions you are required to complete and calculate much time you have for each question. Also note the amount of marks for each section of a question and divide your time accordingly. This time schedule should be adhered to so that you do not lose too much time on one particular question at the expense of others. You should then read through the entire paper identifying questions that you are confident to answer. Before answering questions, ensure that you read the question in its entirety and understand the specific question instructions. For example, if a question asks you to identify three issues, ensure that you give exactly three and that each of the three examples are completely different. With longer questions, ensure that you answer all parts of the question and make sure that your answer sticks to the point of the question and start each question on a new page so as to leave yourself enough room if you want to add any further information to your answer at the end of the exam.

Most written exams can be answered in any order and you should answer the questions in your own preferred order. For electronically marked MCQ and EMI papers take care that you complete the correct corresponding section on the answer sheet. Start with questions that you have identified as knowing the answers to; these early questions will help build confidence and help you relax and settle in to the exam. Completing these questions can also mean that you have more time to spend on the questions that you are unsure of, as answering the easier questions first is generally quicker than answering the ones that require more thought.

Towards the end of the exam, check through your answers, adding anything new you have remembered. Check that you have answered all the required questions and all of the sections for each question you have answered. If you find that you are running out of time with a few questions to answer, prioritise the ones that you answer by the number of marks available for each question.

Methods for setting pass marks

There are many methods for setting the pass marks or cut scores for assessments (Cusimano, 1996). This process is called 'standard setting'. The GMC outlines the required criteria in paragraphs 89 and 90 in *Tomorrow's Doctors* 2009 (Table 5.1). The methods used for standard setting have to be of a defensible standard, fair to students and guarantee that patients receive a good standard of care or competent treatment. Standard setting can fall into categories: fixed pass mark, norm-referenced, combined methods or criterion referenced.

Table 5.1 The General Medical Council's criteria on standards for assessments (GMC, 2009a)

Criteria paragraph 89   There will be systems in place to set appropriate standards for assessments to decide whether students have achieved the curriculum outcomes
Criteria paragraph 90   Assessment criteria will be consistent with the requirements for competence standards set out in disability discrimination legislation. Reasonable adjustments will be provided to help students with disabilities meet these competence standards. Although reasonable adjustments cannot be made to the competence standards themselves, reasonable adjustments should be made to enable a disabled person to meet a competence standard

A fixed pass mark is where a student is required to attain a minimum score on the assessment to pass (e.g. 50 per cent of the marks). This fixed pass mark has the advantage that it is quick and easy for the assessors but has the disadvantage that is it not very defensible and it does not account for any changes in the difficulty of the assessment. Norm-referenced methods identify a set amount of students within the group who pass and fail (e.g. the bottom 10 per cent of students fail the assessment). The advantages of this method are that it identifies the worst-performing students within the group (particularly when there are limited places available such as university entrance or scholarships); the disadvantage is that it does not identify competence in students, it encourages competition and not collaboration and it can lead to declining standards in students.

Combined methods standard setting uses a combination of norm-referenced and fixed pass mark. The Hofstee (Hofstee, 1983) is one example of a combined method. These combined methods use a range of values for the percentage of students failing (e.g. 0–10 per cent) and a range of values for the pass mark (50–70 per cent). These have the advantage that they are easy and give a reasonably fair result for the students. On the down side, they are not that defensible, although they are better than the fixed score and norm-referenced methods for setting the pass mark.

Criterion-referenced standard setting methods are those set using judgements of an expert panel to decide the pass mark. Experts are asked to consider what they would expect the borderline students to achieve within this assessment. The borderline student is one who is not clearly competent nor clearly incompetent. Criterion-based methods have the advantage that they are defensible and fair, but they require a lot of time and resources to complete and some judges find the borderline student a difficult concept to conceptualise.

Case study: Using feedback in practice

While Syed, a foundation year two doctor, is undertaking a paediatric rotation he is asked to put a cannula into a five-year-old child on a ward.

He has struggled with this procedure in the past and had at that time asked to accompany a consultant anaesthetist on a paediatric operating list. The consultant showed him how she gained intravenous access and then gave him constructive feedback on his technique (after having gained consent from the children's carers).

As he prepared the equipment needed for this procedure he reminds himself of what the consultant taught him and especially about how he was not fixing the skin tightly enough to stop the vein from moving. Syed reflects on his experience, thinking how useful the comment made during the teaching was in saving this patient unnecessary pain.

What's the evidence?

The evidence on the effectiveness of medical assessments is immense as it is one of the most important, influential and most widely researched areas of medical education. This is summarised by quotes from two sources:

> Assessment plays a major role in the process of medical education, in the lives of medical students, and in Society by certifying competent physicians who can take care of the public. The very foundation of medical curricula is built around assessment milestones for students.
>
> (Shumway and Harden, 2003)

> *It is impossible to overestimate the importance of assessment. Involvement of teachers in developing assessment procedures is almost certainly the most critical educational task they will undertake. The methods they select and the content they include will have profound effects not only on what students learn but also on how students learn.*
>
> (Newble, 1998)

Chapter summary

This chapter has:

- explained the differences between formative and summative assessments;

- described the common forms of written and practical examinations used during medical training;

- emphasised the importance of feedback provided on assessments;

- given guidance on how students should approach assessments;

- introduced how the pass mark for assessments can be derived.

GOING FURTHER

Exam techniques

- Levin, P (2004) *Sail through Exams!: Preparing for Traditional Exams for Undergraduate and Taught Postgraduates*. Maidenhead: Open University Press.
  This book describes in depth techniques for the taking of different forms of examination.

- Payne, E and Whittaker, L (2006) *Developing Essential Study Skills*. Upper Saddle River, NJ: FT Prentice Hall.
  This book describes different methods for revision and preparation for examinations.

Assessment in medical education

- Schwartz, P and Webb, G (2002) *Assessment: Case Studies, Experience and Practice from Higher Education*. London: Kogan Page.
  This book describes case studies of different assessments detailing the design and method of the assessment but also student perspectives on the assessments.

- Shumway, J and Harden, R (2003) AMEE Guide No. 25: The assessment of learning outcomes for the competent and reflective physician. *Medical Teacher*, 25(6): 569–584.
  This article gives detailed descriptions of the different forms of assessment currently used within medical education.

chapter 6

Teaching and Assessing Communication Skills in Medicine

Gemma Cherry

Achieving your medical degree

This chapter will help you to begin to meet the following requirements of *Tomorrow's Doctors* (GMC, 2009a):

Outcomes 2 – The doctor as a practitioner

Paragraph 15. The graduate will be able to communicate effectively with patients and colleagues in a medical context.

a. Communicate clearly, sensitively and effectively with patients, their relatives or other carers, and colleagues from the medical and other professions, by listening, sharing and responding.
b. Communicate clearly, sensitively and effectively with individuals and groups regardless of their age, social, cultural or ethnic backgrounds or their disabilities, including when English is not the patient's first language.
c. Communicate by spoken, written and electronic methods (including medical records), and be aware of other methods of communication used by patients. The graduate should appreciate the significance of non-verbal communication in the medical consultation.
d. Communicate appropriately in difficult circumstances, such as when breaking bad news, and when discussing sensitive issues, such as alcohol consumption, smoking and obesity.
e. Communicate appropriately with difficult or violent patients.
f. Communicate appropriately with people with mental illness.
g. Communicate appropriately with vulnerable patients.
h. Communicate effectively in various roles, for example, as patient advocate, teacher, manager or improvement leader.

It will also introduce you to the following academic standards as set out in the Quality Assurance Agency's statement for medicine (QAA, 2000):

In relation to interpersonal skills, the graduate will be competent in the following areas of communication:

a. Listening to patients, relatives/carers/partners and other health care professionals
b. Explaining and providing patients and others with adequate information
c. Mediating and negotiating with patients, carers, and colleagues
d. Handling complaints appropriately
e. Liaising with other members of the health care team.

Chapter overview

By reading this chapter you will learn about why communication skills teaching has been introduced into medical curricula and the different ways these skills are taught. Practical examples of teaching practices and exercises for you will provide an in-depth overview of how communication skills are taught and assessed within undergraduate medical curricula. You will be asked to consider why communication is important and which method of teaching communication skills would favour you.

Effective communication in medicine

One cannot not communicate.

(Watzlawick *et al.*, 1967, page 51)

What Watzlawick meant by this is that humans are social creatures; we rely on interactions with other people to maintain our own wellbeing, both physical and mental. Think back to the last time you spoke to or engaged with someone. It is likely that it was very recently as communication, in one form or another, is central to our lives.

ACTIVITY 6.1

Think about who you have communicated with today. Consider your use of speech and language, body language, facial expression, and how the communications made you feel, as well as reasons why you may not have responded to a communication attempt. Has your communication style been different with different people?

For people responsible for providing health care, such as doctors, nurses or social workers, good communication is essential; when doctors use communication skills effectively, both they and their patients benefit. Research has indicated that doctors with good communication skills identify patients' problems more accurately, have greater job satisfaction, less work stress, fewer patient complaints and fewer malpractice claims.

Good communication has also been linked to a number of positive health outcomes for the patient, such as better adherence to treatment, increased likelihood of following advice on behavioural change, less distress, less vulnerability to anxiety and depression, better psychological adjustment and higher satisfaction with their care.

On the other hand, poor communication can also impact on patients' health, and has been shown to result in patients telling their doctors only half of their complaints and concerns; in patients providing little information about their own perceptions of their problems, or the physical, emotional and social impact associated with the problem; and to less than half of all mental illness being recognised. This may lead to doctors prescribing ineffective treatment, or treatment that does not fit with the patient's lifestyle, which may lead to lack of adherence to treatment plans.

The importance of communication as a core competency of undergraduate medical education was first formally recognised in 1993, with the publication of the original *Tomorrow's Doctors* (GMC, 1993). This emphasised the importance of developing skills to interact with patients and colleagues, and resulted in many medical schools investing a great deal in the teaching and assessment of communication skills. In 2002, the ability to communicate competently with patients became a pre-condition of qualification for all health care professionals delivering patient care in the NHS (Department of Health, 2003). Following this, multiple publications have been produced as to how to commission, monitor and provide communication skills education in England. As a result, one of the guiding principles of undergraduate medical education is that the standards set out for communication skills in the GMC's revised *Tomorrow's Doctors* (GMC, 2009a) and the Quality Assurance Agency's (QAA) subject benchmark statement for medicine (QAA, 2000) are embedded within education. These skills are needed for effective communication, and must be present in students upon graduation.

What's the evidence?

Good communication skills expected of health care graduates include the ability to:

- talk to patients, carers and colleagues effectively and clearly, conveying and receiving the intended message;
- enable patients and their carers to communicate effectively;
- listen effectively especially when time is pressured, i.e. skills in engaging and disengaging;
- identify potential communication difficulties and work through solutions;
- understand the differing methods of communication used by individuals;
- understand that there are differences in communication signals between cultures;
- cope in specific difficult circumstances;
- understand how to use and receive non verbal messages given by body language;
- utilise spoken, written and electronic methods of communication;
- know when the information received needs to be passed on to another person/ professional for action;
- know and interpret the information needed to be recorded on patients records, writing discharge letters, copying letters to patients and gaining informed consent;
- recognise the need for further development to acquire specialist skills.

Taken from the Department of Health (2003)

ACTIVITY 6.2

Think about the competencies laid out in the 'What's the evidence?' box. Which would you find difficult? Read up on the specific skills needed for these points. Think about how these may be taught to you in medical school, and which you would need to give particular attention to.

Types of communication in medicine

Communication types range from talking to non-verbal communication using body language, posture and facial expression and listening. Communication can also occur through touch, visually and in written form, and most behaviours communicate something about the person that is doing them. Equally important is non-communication, where a person does not respond to a communication attempt, be it deliberate or unintentional. Five areas of communication are taught and assessed in undergraduate medical curricula: face-to-face communication, telephone communication, written communication, electronic communication and communication through presentation.

Communication skills education in undergraduate medical education

Each medical school teaches communication in slightly different ways, but there are core themes applicable to each medical school. Training in communication skills covers areas such as breaking bad news, consulting patients and relatives, dealing with patients who may be angry, difficult or reluctant, empathy, giving and receiving information and explaining and negotiating (Centre for Change and Innovation, 2003).

There are different methods of integrating communication skills teaching into undergraduate medical education; some schools deliver communication skills as a discrete teaching unit, whereas others integrate communication skills teaching into the curriculum longitudinally, as communication skills are integral to medical practice. A proportion of the curriculum will be allocated for communication skills teaching each year; Hargie *et al.* (2010) found that the overall percentage of total curriculum time allocated to communication skills teaching in each year varied between 0.15 and 5.5 per cent.

In medical school, experiential learning is important for the development of communication skills. Learning usually occurs in small groups.

The following methods of teaching are common to most UK universities teaching medicine.

Hargie and colleagues (Hargie *et al.*, 2010) surveyed all medical schools in the

UK to determine more about communication skills training, and of the 21 that responded, the following results were found.

Role playing

Role playing was used in all schools' teaching of communication skills. This includes role playing within a small group, one-to-one with peers or tutor, or role play with a simulated patient.

Group discussion

This is facilitated by the tutor and allows students to talk about issues and brainstorm within the group. Hargie *et al.* (2010) found that this was reported in 95 per cent of medical schools' undergraduate curricula for teaching of communication skills.

Lectures

Lectures may cover theories of communication skills learning, models or general principles. They may occur as a small group or to the whole year group, and may be interactive. It has been reported that 86 per cent of (responding) medical schools in the UK use lectures as a part of communication skills training (Hargie *et al.*, 2010).

The use of simulated patients

Simulated patients are professional actors who take on the role of a patient in role-play situations. Students are able to practise their communication skills by interviewing the patient, either one-to-one or in front of a small group of peers. Feedback is then given, usually by the patient and the teacher or assessor, and if applicable by peers. The use of simulated patients has increased in the last decade, which is related to two factors: first, it allows students to learn skills in a safe environment before dealing with real patients, and secondly there are now fewer opportunities for students to practise with real patients. (See Chapter 7 for more on simulation.)

Workbooks and homework

These are used throughout sessions to record key points and provide a useful revision aid. Students are able to reflect on their own performance and record feedback from peers, simulated patients and the teacher to later reflect on.

Feedback

This can take the form of tutor-led, peer group-led or simulated patient-led feedback and provides information about the students' communication style. Studies have indicated that effective feedback improves communication.

The use of videoing

Interviews with simulated patients can be videoed to allow for feedback afterwards. Formative objective structured clinical examinations (OSCEs) can also be videoed and re-watched, with feedback given on the strengths and weaknesses of the medical students' communication style provided by the tutor. Videos are a useful platform for self-assessment of communication style.

Ward-based teaching

In later years, teaching of communication skills can take place on wards to allow for overlap between clinical and communication skills. In this setting, real patients are used.

Other teaching methods

Occasionally, seminars and interactive videos may be used to teach communication skills.

Assessment of communication skills

Communication skills are normally assessed as part of OSCEs (see Chapter 5). An OSCE usually comprises a circuit of 5- to 10-minute stations, in which each candidate is examined on a one-to-one basis with one or two trained examiner(s) and either real or, more usually, simulated patients (actors). Each station has a different examiner, as opposed to the traditional method of clinical examinations, in which a candidate would be assigned to an examiner for the entire examination. Candidates rotate through the stations, completing all the stations in one circuit. OSCEs are designed to be standardised, in that all candidates are assessed using the same stations. A timer will go off 1 minute before the end of the time to indicate to you that your time is coming to a close and to conclude your interview. Each station has its own scenario and these will be provided to you prior to the exam.

    Communication skills are assessed in OSCEs using a checklist. These checklists may differ slightly between institutions, but external examiners ensure that all medical schools assess the same communication and interpersonal skills. Students participate in two separate OSCEs – formative and summative. Formative OSCEs take place in January and follow the same format as the summative OSCE. These are assessed, but the assessment is fed back to students to allow them to use it as a practice for the summative OSCE. The formative mark does not count towards passing or failing the year. Feedback is provided from the formative assessment. The summative OSCE takes place at the end of semester two (in May/June).

Case study: Teaching of communication skills at the University of Liverpool

The University of Liverpool has formal teaching in communication skills (called Communication for Clinical Practice, or CCP) in years 1 and 2. Students in their first year are split into groups of approximately nine students, and the course consists of 11 sessions, one every two weeks. This course overlaps with the Clinical Skills Course, and students are taught to demonstrate communication skills while practising clinical procedures with peers or simulated patients. The assessment systems are also similar: both use a formal observed assessment at the end of the second semester.

Sessions consist of group discussion, facilitated by the tutor, interviewing simulated patients and the use of workbooks. Simulated patients attend sessions regularly throughout the course and students practise interviewing them and receiving feedback from the tutor, peer group and patient afterwards. Workbooks are used to record key points and homework, and are useful revision for the OSCE. Sessions also use brainstorms, the use of video cameras to record interviews with simulated patients, and voice recordings on information giving.

Years 3 and 4 contain clinical practice and problem-based learning (PBL) based on the human life cycle, and these are supported by a specialist communication skills unit in year 4. Final examinations are taken at the end of year 4, and year 5 finalises communication skills training with Communication Skills 4 – six half-day tutorials in advanced communication skills. These take place during the community attachment and are assessed as part of the Professional Education and Training Appraisal (PETA) process. Throughout this progression from university to clinical teaching, there is consistent feedback on communication skills.

Key aims of the University of Liverpool's curriculum – communication skills

In the context of social, psychological, ethical, cultural, and physical factors, students will be able to:

1. *listen effectively to patients, consistent with their communication needs, and explore their concerns and expectations;*
2. *recognise and respond appropriately to psychological distress;*
3. *explain diagnosis, prognosis, and treatment in an appropriate way to patients and relatives in terms that they can understand;*

4. *convey bad news sympathetically and to recognize and respond sensitively to the emotion that is generated;*
5. *communicate courteously and effectively with health care colleagues;*
6. *present (and justify) their ideas and evidence orally, in writing, and visually (consistent with Communication Key Skill).*

(University of Liverpool, 2010)

The methods the University uses to develop, practise and assess these skills are summarised in Table 6.1.

Table 6.1 How does the University of Liverpool develop, practise and assess these skills?

Oral communication skills	
Developed through:	Clinical skills
	Communication skills
	Problem-based learning
Practised in:	Clinical practice
	Problem-based learning
Assessed via:	Objective structured clinical examinations
	Liverpool Objective Clinical Assessment System
	Professional Education and Training Appraisal

Written communication skills	
Developed through:	Critical thinking
	Clinical log book
	Elective
	Portfolio
	Special study modules
	Problem-based learning
Practised in:	Critical thinking
	Clinical log book
	Elective
	Portfolio
	Special study modules
	Problem-based learning
Assessed via:	Written examinations
	Professional Education and Training Appraisal
	Critical thinking
	Clinical log book
	Elective
	Portfolio
	Special study modules

Content of communication skills teaching

Much of the training is on *the importance of the medical interview* (or consultation). Within medical education, the tasks and skills required to build relationships are given special emphasis, so that you understand the nature of the doctor's relationship with their patient. Teaching aims to equip you with the skills needed to do this effectively, and in a timely manner. It also aims to show how various tasks within the consultation help you achieve the goal that is in your patients' and your best interests.

There are several main tasks involved in effective communication in consultations. The first is establishing and building a therapeutic relationship with patients. The next steps are the principles of the consultation, such as opening the consultation and setting the agenda. This is crucial given the time constraints of consultations, and allows the patient and yourself to understand the structure of the consultation, eliminating uncertainty. The need to establish, recognise and meet patient needs will be covered also. Needs may include physical, psychological, cultural or religious factors. Other tasks, equally important, include gathering information from the patient, awareness of a patient's world view, and communication skills for conducting a physical examination. Other communication skills include those necessary for explaining diagnoses to patients (and any other individuals present, such as carers or relatives). Integral skills are that of explaining, planning, negotiating, structuring, signposting and prioritising, and these will be fully explained. Often it is necessary to 'skip over' a patient concern that is not directly relevant to the presenting problem due to time issues. Finally you will be educated on ending the interview and setting up the next meeting.

These skills are all discrete, meaning they can occur separately and are not linked, observable, meaning they can be assessed in OSCEs (see above) by examiners, and are specific. Examples include appropriate eye contact, facial expression, balance of open and closed questions, empathic responding, chunking information and checking a patient's understanding.

A large part of what you will be taught in communication skills classes will be about the medical consultation, but not all communication within medicine takes the form of a medical consultation. There are interactions with other health care staff, carers, relatives of patients, and other professional bodies among others, with many different types of communication within those groups. For example, verbal communication, non-verbal communication, communication under time pressures or in an emergency or written communication, in the form of referral letters. Communication between different groups will now be discussed.

Communicating beyond the patient

Doctors are required to communicate with relatives, carers and colleagues from a range of professions, including medical, social work, nursing, and other health backgrounds, law, statutory and voluntary organisations and management groups. All of these interactions rely on basic principles – professionalism, the need to respect others, the importance of evidence-based decision making, the use of reflective practice and medico-legal principles, including respect for patients' confidentiality. In addition, the people that accompany patients to consultations (relatives, carers, advocates, interpreters, etc.) must be considered.

The areas that will be addressed in your undergraduate teaching are communicating with relatives and/or carers, advocates and interpreters, intraprofessional communication and interprofessional communication. Each area has specific challenges associated with it in terms of communication, and these will be addressed fully. For example, you may often be required to communicate with relatives and/or carers either at the patient's request or because the patient does not have the mental capacity to make informed decisions or consent to treatment. Various communication issues will naturally arise in this situation, such as how you will go about including the relative or carer (or 'third party'), how you will ensure that the patient is still able to explain their medical problem freely and without embarrassment or fear with the third party present, how you will maintain the patient's confidentiality, and how you will manage having a third party in the consultation with you.

Case study: Patient confidentiality

Liz was a fifth-year medical student who was on placement at a GP surgery as part of her community placements when she received a telephone call from Mr Angus. Mr Angus was concerned about his wife, who had recently been in to see Liz. Mrs Angus had been very forgetful lately and Mr Angus was concerned that she may have Alzheimer's. He had asked his wife what the doctor had said when she got back from her appointment, but Mrs Angus couldn't remember properly. Mr Angus wanted to know what Liz and her GP supervisor had thought of his wife's forgetfulness, and what they should do about it.

Mrs Angus had mentioned to Liz that she had not brought her husband to the surgery with her because he gets very angry at her for forgetting things, and she was scared of his reaction if he found out that she was to be referred onto Alzheimer's services.

Liz explained to Mr Angus that she could not discuss his wife's case on the telephone with him, and advised him to make an appointment to see the GP with his wife.

ACTIVITY 6.3

Think about what you would have done in Liz's situation. How would you have been sure that it was Mrs Angus's husband that you were talking to? How would you be able to find out what Mr Angus already knew without breaking Mrs Angus's confidence? In what situation would you have discussed Mrs Angus with her husband?

Another difficult situation may be communicating with advocates and interpreters. Advocates are people who are there on the request of the patient, and who present their views. You will need to learn skills to work with advocates effectively, as well as the communication skills needed when liaising with interpreters. Such skills involve maintenance of confidentiality, definition of the parameters of their role and how to work within cultural and practical constraints. You can see that some of these skills have already been mentioned in the key themes of communication skills training discussed earlier.

Intraprofessional communication means communicating within a health care team. You will need to write patient charts, as well as hand over to staff after a shift, write referral letters, discuss issues (both patient and non-patient related) with colleagues, as well as many other communicative skills. The curriculum will cover the need for clear and comprehensible clinical communication, both written and oral, as well as issues around handover and ward round presentations. You'll also be taught skills to help you to be appropriately assertive when working with colleagues. As a doctor, you have a responsibility, dictated by the General Medical Council (GMC), to maintain safety in the health care environment, so you will be informed how to express your concerns to peers or colleagues about their performance. It is also important that you know how complaints from colleagues, patients or relatives are processed, and the impact of being the subject of a complaint or making an error.

You will also be taught the importance of interpersonal communication – the ability to understand the roles that other team members play, how to promote effective collaboration and communicate to ensure that care is continued from different environments, such as from primary care (GP surgeries) to secondary care (the hospital). This includes principles of data sharing and confidentiality associated with this.

Your communication skills teaching will help you to learn skills to manage these situations effectively.

What's the evidence?

'Several studies show that a large proportion of complaints against doctors arise from problems or difficulties in communication' (Halperin, 2000). It would seem then that there are still improvements to be made in terms of the abilities of doctors to communicate effectively with their patients.

Based on this growing evidence, medical education governing bodies embraced clinical communication as a vital component of their various curricula. An excerpt from the General Medical Council's (GMC) Tomorrow's Doctors document, relating to undergraduate medical education in the UK (General Medical Council, 2009) states that communication and consultation skills are part of 'doctor as practitioner' and competence in this area must be demonstrated.

(Laidlaw and Hart, 2011)

Chapter summary

This chapter has explained how:

- communication is an integral part of clinical practice, and is a core competency as laid out by the GMC (2009a);

- clinical communication involves communicating with patients, their relatives/carers/advocates, other members of the health care team and other professionals;

- communication takes many forms, such as spoken, written and non-verbal;

- communication skills training is integrated within undergraduate medical education;

- communication skills training and use of varied styles of feedback will help you to identify areas in which you need practice and to practise these skills in a safe environment;

- communication is assessed in undergraduate medical education;

- good communication can improve patient care.

GOING FURTHER

- Lloyd, M and Bor, R (2009) *Communication Skills for Medicine*. New York: Churchill Livingstone Inc.
  This book provides a really good overview of communication skills for medical students. It contains lots of case studies and practical examples.

- Silverman, J, Kurtz, SM and Draper, J (2005) *Skills for Communicating with Patients*. Oxford: Radcliffe Publishing.
  A good overview of the skills that are needed when communicating with patients.

chapter 7

Simulation

Michael Moneypenny

Achieving your medical degree

This chapter will help you to begin to meet the following requirements of *Tomorrow's Doctors* (GMC, 2009):

Outcomes 2 – The doctor as a practitioner

The graduate will be able to:

13. Carry out a consultation with a patient
14. Diagnose and manage clinical presentations
15. Communicate effectively with patients and colleagues in a medical context
16. Provide immediate care in medical emergencies
18. Carry out practical procedures safely and effectively.

Outcomes 3 – The doctor as a professional

The graduate will be able to:

22. Learn and work effectively within a multiprofessional team.

Chapter overview

Professor David Gaba defined simulation as a technique: 'to replace or amplify real experiences with guided experiences that evoke or replicate substantial aspects of the real world in a fully interactive manner' (Gaba, 2004). Simulation encompasses a wide range of techniques, from part-task trainers to simulated patients to high-fidelity simulation suites. This chapter will explore what Professor Gaba's quote means and how and why simulation is being used in medical education. The role of simulation in teaching and assessment is set to expand markedly and, although simulation has many advantages, it also has limitations. The informed medical student will be aware of these limitations and know how to make full use of the learning opportunities that this rapidly evolving technique provides.

After reading this chapter you will be able to:

- discuss what is meant by the term 'simulation' in the context of medical education;
- appreciate why and how simulation is being increasingly used in both undergraduate and postgraduate teaching and assessment;
- compare the benefits and drawbacks of using simulation;
- understand how to make the most of the opportunities for learning provided by simulation.

Simulation is a technique

As Gaba states, simulation is a technique, method or strategy for learning, teaching and assessing. Simulation is therefore more than the physical reproduction of a part of anatomy or a clinical setting; it is instead a method of attempting to create a mind-set within the person interacting with the simulation that the simulation is 'real'.

Within medical education, simulation encompasses a wide range of techniques and tools. These include the following:

- Simulating a clinical interaction with a fellow medical student or a simulated patient (actor), where you are the doctor and he or she is the patient.

- Simulating a scenario, such as a general practice visit on a computer.

- Simulating a part of anatomy, such as a model (part-task trainer) for performing rectal examinations.

- Simulating a trauma scenario in a purpose-built simulation suite where you are a member of a multiprofessional team looking after a mannequin which can reproduce signs of shock.

Although you may read about simulation being defined as low or high fidelity, these terms are not particularly useful. High fidelity implies high-cost simulation suite-based work, and low fidelity tends to refer to models of limbs or parts of anatomy. However there is a large grey area between these two extremes. Also, simulation involving simulated patients (actors) or computer-based simulation is difficult to classify as high or low fidelity.

What's the evidence?

Numerous studies have shown that those who perform a skill using simulation go on to perform this skill more quickly and with fewer mistakes than those who did not have the benefit of simulation practice (Naik et al., 2001; Fried et al., 2004). These findings seem self-evident and probably reflect your own experience; the more you practise something, the better you become. The caveat is, of course, that you must practise the correct technique, which is where the guided experience becomes important to point out mistakes of omission or commission. Repeated practice of the wrong technique means you will become very good at performing it the wrong way!

In medical education, therefore, simulation is a way of learning or assessing which involves reproducing a real experience. The rationale for the increase in popularity of simulation is discussed in the following section.

Simulation replaces real experiences with guided experiences

Simulation has been used for centuries in the military domain, with units of soldiers practising defensive and offensive formations and manoeuvres against a simulated enemy. More recently, simulation has been introduced into the aviation industry and is now pervasive throughout this high-risk field. The use of simulation in medicine is somewhat more recent and the increase in use and interest in the past few years has several causes, including:

- an increase in the number of medical students with the demand for patients presenting with a given pathology outstripping the supply;

- an increase in patient autonomy and the need for informed consent with a move away from the idea that it is acceptable to risk harming patients for training purposes;

- the development of synthetic materials and computer technology which allow accurate reproduction of human anatomy and physiology;

- a reform in medical education with a focus on whether medical undergraduates and postgraduates are able to perform essential skills as opposed to writing or talking about them.

In his 2008 annual report, the Chief Medical Officer (CMO) for England wrote: 'Simulation training in all its forms will be a vital part of building a safer health care system' (Chief Medical Officer, 2009, page 55). This was the latest in a long line of opinions and advice that the medical community should be using simulation more frequently. For many specialties, the future of the application of learned skills will be simulation on a part-task trainer, followed by simulation in a purpose-built simulation suite, and only then will doctors be allowed to perform on patients.

The increase in the use of simulation has several perceived advantages. These include:

- avoidance of the potential to harm patients;

- repetitive, guided practice leading to familiarisation and mastery of a skill or behaviour;

- standardisation of assessments on tasks which are either rarely seen or would be unethical to reproduce in patients, such as the treatment of anaphylaxis or drowning.

ACTIVITY 7.1

Imagine you are the course director for a medical school with 300 students per year. You need to show the GMC and the public that your medical students are fit to practise. One way of proving this is by assessing medical students' skills in

---

practical procedures and communication. You think that medical students should be able to appropriately examine a female breast and discuss their findings with the patient. You would like to assess the students in their ability to carry out these skills. Consider:

- How would you objectively assess 300 medical students before the advent of simulation?
- What impact would the use of a prosthetic breast make?
- How could you improve on the use of a prosthetic breast?

Before the advent of simulation, there was no method for objectively assessing an entire year's cohort of medical students on a practical procedure such as breast examination. Although one may have been able to assess every medical student at some point in his or her training, it would have been logistically difficult and inappropriate and painful for the patient for every medical student to examine the same breast. With the replacement of the real experience with a guided experience such as a prosthetic breast, the discomfort to the patient is removed and the part to be examined can be standardised. For breast examination, a lump of a defined size, consistency and position can be placed in the prosthetic breast and the students can be assessed on their examination skills and ability to accurately describe their findings.

All this talk of assessment may lead to activation of your sympathetic nervous system (tachycardia, sweating, tachypnoea, etc.). This should not be the case, as the section heading talks about a guided experience. This may refer to the internal guide within you (i.e. 'Am I doing this right?'). More often, however, it refers to an external guide who assesses or, to use friendlier terms, evaluates or watches your performance. This guide can then give you feedback on your technique and ability to describe your findings because you are performing the technique on a standardised model. In addition, because this is a prosthetic model, you can carry out as many performances as you wish until your technical skill is practised and fluid.

A recent development that aims to improve on the use of disembodied parts of anatomy for training and assessment is melding the part to be examined with a simulated patient. In the breast examination example, a prosthetic breast can be attached to a simulated patient and the seams covered up by a gown. This allows the medical student to gain informed consent, perform the examination and discuss his or her findings with the patient in a manner which more accurately reflects real life.

Finally, some centres have reported the use of simulated patients who are willing to allow intimate examinations to be performed on them (Hendrickx *et al.*, 2006). Although there are clear benefits in terms of feedback regarding technique, the loss of standardisation and the inability to reproduce pathology mean that these willing volunteers are unlikely to become the norm.

The expansion in the use of simulation is not confined to undergraduate medical education. A variety of simulation techniques (simulated patients, part-task trainers and mannequins) are now used in postgraduate training and assessment. For example, the UK Royal College of Anaesthetists uses simulated patients to assess communication skills and a mannequin to assess competency in the treatment of anaesthetic emergencies in the Primary Fellowship (FRCA) exams. This means that the experience you gain at an undergraduate level is invaluable when faced with similar simulation techniques later on in your career.

We have explored why simulation is useful in both undergraduate and postgraduate assessment and education. It allows assessments to be standardised, every examinee can be asked to perform the same procedure or task on the same object, without the potential for harming a patient if errors are made. However, there are also limitations and disadvantages which are discussed in the following section.

Simulation replicates the real world

Simulation, by definition, is not reality; rather it is a reproduction of elements of reality. Simulation design involves deciding which elements of reality are required to replicate the real world in sufficient detail for the assessment of learning objectives.

ACTIVITY 7.2

One of the arguments made by critics of simulation is that simulation, such as breaking bad news to a simulated patient, is not 'real'. Thus, the argument goes, assessing how a medical student acts in such a setting cannot and should not be extrapolated to how the same student would perform in 'the real world'. What are your thoughts on this view?

Read the following papers:

Reznick, RK, Blackmore, D and Cohen, R (1993) An objective structured clinical examination for the licentiate of the Medical Council of Canada: from research to reality. *Academic Medicine*, 68(Suppl): S4–S6.

Wass, V, Jones, R and Van der Vleuten, C (2001) Standardized or real patients to test clinical competence? The long case revisited. *Medical Education*, 35: 321–325.

Have these papers made a difference to your opinions?

One of the recent developments in simulation is the use of mobile simulation suites. Examples include the mobile simulation platform used in Scotland (Clinical Skills Managed Educational Network, 2009) and the 'inflatable simulation suite' used by Professor Kneebone and his colleagues from Imperial College London (ICL) (Kneebone *et al.*, 2010). The latter is a model for 'good enough' simulation. The anaesthetic machine in the operating suite is actually a poster of an anaesthetic machine. The group from ICL have found that the surgical team do not care or seem to notice that the anaesthetic machine is not real because they become focused on the task they are performing. This is an important point to note regarding your own experience with simulation. What at first may seem a very unrealistic setting, such as a classroom, can, with the use of a few essential props and adoption of roles by the participants, be turned into a ward or emergency medicine department.

The decision about how realistic the simulation needs to be is made on the basis of factors such as cost, time, availability of staff, equipment and learning objectives. Sometimes this decision is a poor one and there is a disconnect between the required and actual level of simulation. In the classroom example above, one could imagine a scenario where one of the participants performs the role of a collapsed patient. The other participants might then carry out an airway, breathing, circulation and disability (ABCD) examination. This would not seem unrealistic if the learning objectives were to assess candidates' ability to perform an ABCD exam. However this would not be the case if the learning objectives were to assess candidates' ability to perform cardiopulmonary resuscitation (CPR). Asking the candidates to pretend to perform CPR on their colleague may result in the breakdown of the simulation and a failure to meet those learning objectives. One of the disadvantages of simulation then is that it may at times not be real enough.

Case study: Meeting learning objectives

Louise is a fourth-year medical student who has always had trouble remembering the exact steps that she needs to follow during a cardio-vascular examination. Although she is given opportunities to practise this skill on the wards, she feels embarrassed when she makes mistakes. She also doesn't feel comfortable checking she is doing the right thing by looking at the practical skills book in front of the patient.

Louise has read about how simulation mannequins can be used to practise skills. Because she doesn't have easy access to a simulation suite, she decides instead to practise her skills on a pillow. Although she feels a bit foolish to begin with, Louise practises her cardiovascular exam once or twice a night. She makes sure she is doing it correctly and not missing any steps by reviewing her performance from her clinical skills book.

By the time of her objective structured clinical examination (OSCE) Louise's cardiovascular examination is confident, fluid and second-nature to her. She passes the cardiovascular station with flying colours.

A corollary of this lack of sufficient equipment or staff to support the simulation is the use of superfluous or overly complicated equipment. The more complicated the equipment, the more likely it is that it will malfunction during the simulation, which may result in the loss of the learning opportunity.

Much of the discussion so far on how simulation is used to replicate the real world has focused on equipment and technical issues. Another aspect, which may play a much greater part in the success or failure of a simulation, is the human element. This refers to the people who are helping (or hindering) your simulation experience: the simulated patients, your colleagues and the faculty.

Where simulated patients (actors) are being used, they may turn out to be poor at performing their role. For example they may allow their responses and willingness to divulge information to be dependent on whether or not they like the person being assessed.

Many of the simulation episodes using mannequins require a team of participants to manage the 'patient'. This means that nursing students and medical students may be required to perform their respective roles. This multiprofessional simulation can help you learn how to work effectively as a team.

The third human element consists of the faculty who are responsible for designing and running the simulations. In fact, many of the equipment and environment problems we have discussed so far can be mitigated or avoided by a dedicated and trained faculty. A well-informed faculty will ensure that simulated patients are trained and perform their roles objectively. They will design scenarios that meet the learning objectives and use the correct, well-maintained equipment. Lastly, the capable faculty will ensure that they provide useful, timely and helpful feedback to the candidates who are being assessed.

The final potential disadvantage to using simulation is therefore its reliance on a guide who will ensure that the simulation is appropriate and the practice provided is of benefit to the learner.

Table 7.1 summarises the advantages and disadvantages of simulation, while the following section explains how you can make the most of the opportunities that simulation provides.

Table 7.1 The advantages and disadvantages of simulation

Advantages	Disadvantages
Repeatable	Requires suspension of disbelief
Standardised	Equipment may malfunction
Safe (for learners and patients)	May not be realistic enough or overly complicated
Allows training for rare events	Requires trained faculty

Simulation is interactive

Every encounter in which simulation is used allows you to have one of two mindsets. You can either attempt to immerse yourself in the simulated encounter and suspend your disbelief, or you can remain outside the simulated encounter and refrain from fully participating.

Every simulation will require a degree of interaction between you and the simulation in order for you to get the most out of the learning opportunity. Scenarios taking place in a simulation suite are frequently realistic enough that you do not need to force yourself into thinking that they are 'real'. By the same token, scenarios which involve isolated body parts, such as urinary catheterisation, do not require

---

ACTIVITY 7.3

Try out the following activity with one or more friends. One person should play the role of a simulated patient attending their GP surgery with a concern such as headaches. The other person should play the role of the GP. If there are additional participants they can watch the interaction. First, try the scenario with the mindset of refusing to believe in the simulation (i.e. this is not a real patient, he/she does not have a headache and you are having to pretend to take a history etc.). Next, try the same scenario but this time suspend your disbelief: this is a real patient who is coming to you with headaches, they could be benign or sinister, organic or psychological, etc.

Afterwards, discuss with your colleague how they felt when you did not immerse yourself in the simulation compared to when you did. Did they notice a difference? Discuss how you felt when you suspended your disbelief. Were your clinical, communication and diagnostic skills challenged when you bought into the simulation? Which mindset do you think is more likely to benefit your learning? If there were additional participants, discuss with them how they would rate your communication and clinical skills in the two scenarios.

---

you to pretend that they are real. However, you may have difficulty immersing yourself in simulations which involve your colleagues playing a role or those in which a simulated patient is used. It is not unusual to hear medical students complain that they feel as if they are having to act a part, such as a concerned doctor when breaking bad news, in front of another person who is also just acting a part (i.e. the simulated patient).

If you are one of those medical students then you may be reassured that you are not alone in finding it difficult to interact with a simulation or simulated patient. The key to success is to continue to practise. The more you practise the less awkward you will feel and the more you will be able to concentrate on the information you are meant to be gathering rather than the realism of the simulation.

What's the evidence?

A requirement for the use of a training or assessment technique is that it is acceptable to those being trained or assessed. In this context, simulation performs very well. A range of surveys have shown that students enjoy simulation work and that they think it is both realistic and useful (Gordon et al., 2001; Weller, 2004). I am frequently approached by final-year medical students who tell me they wish they had had more simulation earlier on in their undergraduate career.

The following section will provide you with some advice on how to make simulation work for you.

Using simulation to help you learn

There are three main strategies which you can use to ensure maximum learning from your simulation experiences. The first is to practise the skills required of you within the simulation, the second is to practise the mindset that is required of you and the third is to reflect on your performance at the end of every simulation session.

First, therefore, make use of all the simulation tools available to you. Practise on the models, preferably with a friend who can check your performance against the required standard, until your practice is fluid and easy. In my role as a medical student OSCE examiner it is evident who has repeatedly practised the procedure and who is only doing it for the second or third time. If you are competent and confident with the technical skill you will be less nervous during the exam (which will be noted by the examiner and any simulated patient) and you will be able to allocate more of your mental resources to coming up with differential diagnoses and putting the simulated patient at ease.

Second, practise 'buying into' the simulation. Some find this task easier than others and you may have to work hard at this at first. By immersing yourself in the simulation, however, you are more likely to perform as you would in reality and you will therefore gain the most from your experience. Also, the person who is assessing you will be able to provide you with feedback on your skill and behaviour rather than having to focus on your inability or unwillingness to interact with the simulation.

Finally, use any feedback you get and your own view on how well you did in order to reflect on what you did well and what you could have done better. Use the lessons you have learnt from your reflection to improve your performance next time.

In the final section we will consider how the role of simulation in the medical field might evolve.

The future of simulation in health care

It remains unclear how simulation will develop in the future. There are a number of factors which will influence its use in training and assessment, including cost, apathy and lack of training.

ACTIVITY 7.4

Spend a couple of minutes thinking about how simulation might develop in the future. Then please read the following papers:

Bradley, P (2006) The history of simulation in medical education and possible future directions. *Medical Education*, 40: 254–262.

Gaba, D (2004) The future vision of simulation in health care. *Quality and Safety in Health Care*, 13(Suppl 1): i2–i10.

Now that you have read those papers, what do you think simulation might be used for in the future?

In his paper, Gaba (2004) talks about a holodeck (as seen in 'Star Trek') as the zenith of simulation technology. In the holodeck, participants interact with sophisticated holograms which are indistinguishable from real people. Although this level of artificial reality is unlikely to be achieved in the near future, advances in simulation design will undoubtedly result in an increase in the realism of the technologies.

A parallel strand, and one in which much research is still required, is the development of the non-physical aspects of simulation. Questions such as the best way of debriefing participants, the ideal ratio between simulated and 'real' clinical care and the most appropriate method for guiding simulated learning, remain unanswered. Dismukes and colleagues (2006) suggest that the debrief is the key aspect of the entire simulation experience, so the importance of these psychological issues should not be underestimated.

Simulation is being increasingly used in both undergraduate and postgraduate training and assessments, including the revalidation of consultants. The role of simulation will expand further until it will be expected that you will have performed and familiarised yourself with a technique before you are allowed to 'practise' on a patient. Used appropriately, it is a powerful technique that will make you a better doctor. By putting yourself at ease in a simulated environment through repeated practice and buy-in as early as possible in your medical career, you will reap the benefits and, perhaps more importantly, so will your patients.

Chapter summary

In this chapter we covered:

- what is meant by the term simulation;
- why simulation is being used in teaching and assessment;
- the advantages and disadvantages of simulation;
- why you must interact with the simulation to benefit from it;
- how to use simulation-based learning to your advantage;
- the future of simulation in health care.

GOING FURTHER

- Bokken, L, Rethans, J-J, Scherpbier, AJJA and van der Vleuten, CPM (2008) Strengths and weaknesses of simulated and real patients in the teaching of skills to medical students: a review. *Simulation in Healthcare*, 3: 161–169.

This paper looks at how simulated and real patients are of use in teaching medical undergraduates. There are numerous references to other work on this topic.

- Maran, NJ and Glavin, RJ (2003) Low- to high-fidelity simulation – a continuum of medical education? *Medical Education*, 37(Suppl. 1): 22–28.
This paper gives an overview of the types of simulations in use and how they are supported by current educational theory.

chapter 8

Student Selected Components (SSCs)

Simon Watmough

Achieving your medical degree

This chapter will help you to begin to meet the following requirements of *Tomorrow's Doctors* (GMC, 2009a):

Outcomes 1 – The doctor as a scholar and a scientist

The graduate will be able to:

12. Apply scientific method and approaches to medical research.

   (a) Critically appraise the results of relevant diagnostic, prognostic and treatment trials and other qualitative and quantitative studies as reported in the medical and scientific literature.
   (b) Formulate simple relevant research questions in biomedical science, psychosocial science or population science, and design appropriate studies or experiments to address the questions.
   (c) Apply findings from the literature to answer the questions raised by specific clinical problems.
   (d) Understand the ethical and governance issues involved in medical research.

Standards for the delivery of teaching, learning and assessment:

96. The purpose of student selected components (SSCs) is the intellectual development of students through exploring in-depth a subject of their choice.
97. SSC learning outcomes must be mapped to outcomes in *Tomorrow's Doctors* and contained within the assessment blueprint for the programme, thus helping to make SSCs transparently relevant and clarify how SSCs contribute to the programme.

Chapter overview

A fundamental skill for all doctors to maintain and develop is to engage in areas which interest them, develop research skills and keep up to date with the latest treatments and developments in medicine. One way to do this is to develop self-directed research skills through researching a topic of interest and then writing up the results of this research into a coherent paper during an SSC.

After reading this chapter you will be able to:
- understand why SSCs are an important component of today's undergraduate medical curricula;
- gain a knowledge of the different type of SSCs;
- understand why the skills SSCs will develop are vital for a doctor's future career.

Student selected components

Student selected components (SSCs) were recommended by the General Medical Council (GMC) in the first edition of *Tomorrow's Doctors*. As we have already seen in Chapter 2, *Tomorrow's Doctors* recommends that medical curricula should have a core curriculum supported by a series of SSCs. The GMC has been careful not to use the term 'options' for these components so both students and medical schools don't consider that they are in any way an optional part of the curriculum (Murdoch-Eaton *et al.*, 2004). It was originally recommended by the GMC that approximately one-third of a curriculum was to be selected by medical students. In the original *Tomorrow's Doctors* they were known as special study modules (SSMs), which is how some institutions in the UK refer to them today, but by the second version of *Tomorrow's Doctors* the GMC rephrased the term as student selected components.

Prior to these recommendations the only real student selected components were electives and there is a section about these on pages 84 and 85. The latest *Tomorrow's Doctors* stipulates that SSCs must be 'an integral part of the curriculum', enabling students to demonstrate mandatory competences while allowing choice in studying an area of particular interest. The curriculum must allow for at least 10 per cent of course time for this, although many medical schools offer more time than this and students should have freedom of choice to choose from a wide range of SSCs to allow them to explore areas that interest them and to take responsibility for their own learning.

The introduction of SSCs reflected trends in the medical education community world wide (Riley, 2009). The World Federation for Medical Education (WFME) produced a document called *Global Standards for Quality Improvement* (WFME, 2003), which highlights the importance of 'optional content' in medical curricula. Some countries go further than this to encourage students to develop research skills. In Germany, for example, medical school graduates practise medicine but cannot call themselves 'doctor' until they have completed a thesis. The University of Melbourne has recently introduced a four-year Doctor of Medicine course for graduates taught at master's level. North American medical schools have had graduate entry programmes for many years and now many medical schools in the UK offer graduate entry programmes. SSCs are therefore useful for students who do not have the experience of a prior degree to gain the research experience that some of their peers may already have.

It is also important to remember that research as an undergraduate is nothing new. Charles Best was a medical student working as an assistant to Dr Frederick Banting and played a major role in helping to discover insulin. This is not to say you are expected to make major new discoveries as a student! However, you can develop research skills as an undergraduate and SSCs can help you achieve this.

In 1993, the GMC suggested that the majority of SSCs offered by medical schools should be based on subjects directly related to medicine, for example laboratory based or clinical, biological or behavioural, research orientated or descriptive. However, the GMC did not stipulate that they should be exclusively restricted to these areas and SSCs can also include, for instance, maths and physics, social sciences and philosophy or even languages, literature or the history of medicine. The University of Sheffield, for example, in 2010 offered SSCs in the following areas: history of medicine, critical analysis, communicating health education, research attachments in biomedical, population, behavioural or clinical sciences, clinical attachments, public health, 'topics beyond medicine' and applied scientific principles in psychiatry, neurology or medicine for older people (University of Sheffield, 2010). This ties in with the philosophy espoused in all versions of *Tomorrow's Doctors* that students should embrace disciplines outside medicine.

Although medical schools have a great deal of flexibility in the way they interpret *Tomorrow's Doctors*, many of the core curricula within medical schools are quite prescriptive; students will have to attend certain clinical skills and science classes and many attachments in medicine, surgery or the community will be compulsory. A criticism of SSCs is that it is not always possible to match students with their choices. However, as it is not always possible to match student choice with availability of convenors, many universities allow students to develop their own SSCs and then approach a convenor to supervise them.

Also, as the number of medical specialties has increased in recent years there are more and more specialties and subspecialties that are not covered in undergraduate medical education. Therefore, SSCs are a good way of giving students exposure to smaller specialties which you would not necessarily experience as undergraduates – for example, clinical genetics, radiology and maxillofacial surgery.

Skills you will develop while undertaking SSCs

One thing that is common to the vast majority of SSCs is allowing you to develop the skills for accessing and critically assessing research. A study has concluded that greater student input into SSCs can have a positive impact, notably in assisting students' self-directed learning skills (Murphy *et al.*, 2009). Although not all doctors will undertake research, they will still need skills to keep up to date with the latest literature as advances in treatments are made. Also, as Chapters 1 and 2 have highlighted, it is not possible for students to cover all aspects of clinical medicine as undergraduates. While all SSCs at different medical schools are slightly different in the way they are organised and assessed, there are purposes common to all SSC programmes (Murdoch-Eaton *et al.*, 2004).

These are:

- to extend experiences and interests beyond the core curriculum;
- to provide opportunity to choose and pursue topics of personal, academic and vocational interest;
- to apply and develop skills in research/evaluation of the scientific basis of practice;
- to enhance personal and professional development.

There are also common expected learning activities across SSCs where students should be provided with opportunities to apply and enhance a range of skills, including:

- information gathering (using for example, library and electronic databases);
- IT skills (web searching, patient information systems, log books, portfolios);
- critical analysis and review (criticise, evaluate and interpret evidence from all sources and exposure to evidence-based medicine and audit);
- research methodologies (exposure to both quantitative and qualitative methodologies) and participate in research by themselves or in a team (i.e. with the SSC convenor).

Different types of SSC

Institutions offer different kinds of SSCs to students. These are some of the typical types of SSC on offer to students.

Structured review SSCs

These allow students to undertake a literature review on a certain area using at least one electronic search engine. They are then expected to discuss the literature, giving a background to the study, and critically appraise the literature in the discussion before drawing conclusions, summarising the main findings, the methodological strengths and weakness and offering areas for future study.

Survey-based SSCs

These aim to familiarise students with the process of undertaking primary research, including developing a research proposal, data analysis and writing up the results. The data can be qualitative or quantitative and, if necessary, ethical approval will have to be sought for the SSC.

Scenario one

John undertakes an SSC carrying out a literature search (or structured review) about the reasons why students may or may not undertake a career in academic medicine. He realised this is an area which interests him so he approaches his convenor to ask if for his next SSC he could undertake a research project (or survey-based SSC) asking his peers what their career intentions are and whether they would be interested in a career in academic medicine. He draws up a questionnaire which is sent to all the students in his year. He manages to publish the results in a medical education journal. Having this publication on his CV is a major factor in him gaining a place on an Academic Foundation Programme after he graduated.

Interpretative-based SSCs

These are aimed to allow students to analyse and interpret data and can be undertaken with either quantitative or qualitative data. For quantitative studies the student should focus on numerics, which, for example, can include analysis of audit data or re-analysis of collected data or involve the students distributing a questionnaire of their own. A qualitative study may involve a review of the published results of interviews or focus groups or carrying out interviews or focus groups themselves.

Laboratory-based SSCs

These could either involve carrying out experiments during the SSC (if time permits and the facilities are available) or they can involve undertaking a structured review based on laboratory methodology and activities or integrating practical laboratory elements alongside a structured review.

Case-based SSCs

In these, students interpret patient-related information in the context of current literature. This could include treatment outcomes, management of illnesses and the pathology of diseases.

Scenario two

Jeremy has always been fascinated by pathology since he was a child after watching television programmes involving forensic pathologists. He undertook an SSC with a forensic pathologist and as part of this placement he undertook an interpretive SSC reviewing studies on the commonest criminal autopsies in the UK. He really enjoyed this placement and during this he came into contact with other branches of pathology. For his next SSC he took a case-based SSC in histopathology reviewing the literature surrounding diseases. Not only did he realise that there was much more to pathology than just using a microscope, but he also realised that histopathologists work closely with a whole range of other clinical specialties and have an active involvement in patient care. He is now considering this as a career choice.

ACTIVITY 8.1

Think of an area of medicine that particularly interests you. Find out more about that interest. How would you find out more information about that specific topic? How difficult was it to find any information about it? Did you find any conflicting information from different sources?

Relevance of SSCs after graduation

As well as gaining literature searching, research and critical evaluation skills which will help you in your undergraduate degree, SSCs will help you gain skills which you will need for the rest of your career and enhance your CV.

Research skills

All doctors need to keep up to date with progress in medicine, such as the development of new therapies and new drugs and the evidence base for these. Also, doctors are expected to keep up to date with NHS guidelines and procedures which change regularly. The majority of doctors are expected to write reports for their departments in hospitals and publish papers in peer-reviewed journals. Many SSCs have strict criteria over the way they should be presented and have word limits, mirroring the criteria which journals stipulate for papers to be published. These would also be essential skills for any student thinking of a career in academic medicine. Publishing in peer-reviewed journals can help a doctor be successful when applying for competitive posts and the skills needed to write papers for publication are practised while undertaking SSCs.

Developments in each medical specialty and constant changes in the structure and expectations of doctors by the NHS require all doctors to be able to search and review literature efficiently and effectively. The term 'literature' includes books, different types of journals, including e-journals and 'grey' literature such as papers and presentations at conferences. Through SSCs, students should become familiar with literature search engines such as Medline, and different search engines can be used for different topics.

Audits

Nearly all doctors will undertake audits during their careers (an audit being evidence collected for actions or treatments which can improve patient care or safety in a localised setting, often undertaken in a ward or department or across a hospital) and SSCs offer the opportunity to undertake audits.

Enhancing your CV

Having an audit or publication on a CV as an undergraduate can help with applications for training posts. Chapter 11 on careers will illustrate why CVs are important and why it is vital that students start thinking about their careers, even as undergraduates. Well-researched and presented SSCs can also help students gain honours degrees, which can be a big advantage on a CV for your medical career.

ACTIVITY 8.2

The following three references give details of their SSCs on the website of three different UK medical schools. Read through them and notice how similar their objectives are, despite being written by different medical schools and how they meet the GMC guidelines on SSCs. Notice how they are arranged at different times in each course and the assessment criteria.

University of Dundee (2010) www.dundee.ac.uk/medschool/mbchb. Dundee MBChB programme.

University of Newcastle (2010) http://ssm.ncl.ac.uk/stage4/home/ Student Selected Components.

University of Sheffield (2010) www.sheffield.ac.uk/aume/curriculum_dev/ssc.html Student Selected Components.

How do they work in practice?

Case study: University of Liverpool

SSCs are known as special study modules (SSMs) in Liverpool and students have to take six SSMs from years 1 to 4. Five take place over a four-week period and one takes place one day a week over a four-month period to mimic the time doctors, particularly doctors in training, may have to work on research while undertaking clinical duties for the rest of their time. 'They are designed to encourage diversity of approach and to give students the choice and opportunities to explore particular interests while developing intellectual and practical skills essential for scientific and medical practice' (University of Liverpool, 2010).

A list of all the topics available and list of convenors is made available to all students for each SSM at Liverpool. Each SSC has a short abstract where the convenor indicates what the aim of the SSC is and what the student is expected to learn undertaking this SSC. Students write down up to five topics in preference and where possible are allocated their preferred choice.

The students at the start of each SSC meet with their convenor and at the meeting they agree a learning contract which they both sign where they discuss how the SSC will progress. At this stage the student and convenor agree to meet up in about a week to check there are no problems finding the relevant literature. Often between four and eight students are allocated to a convenor for an SSM and the initial meetings may take place in a group so students can share ideas with each other as well as the convenor. Further contact may take place via emails or phone before the end of the SSM or if it is a laboratory-based SSM regular meetings in the lab may be arranged. Also, the students have to include a timetable of their work when they hand in their SSMs and have it verified by their convenor.

The SSMs are marked according to set criteria which are clearly laid out, and serve as a basis for assessment of student performance. These seven objectives aim to enable each student:

- to explain why the study was needed;
- to explain what the study was expected to achieve and the extent to which this was met;
- to outline what you did;
- to outline what you found;
- to explain what that means;
- to explain the relevance of the findings to current evidence-base and indicate possible future application;

- to present the study in a well-organised, formal way (including the logical flow of concepts, grammar, typography and referencing).

All seven criteria are marked accordingly as either unsatisfactory, fair, good or excellent and the SSCs are marked by the convenor and a second marker who have to agree the final mark. All SSMs have to conform to the 'Vancouver' referencing system and be 3000 words long ±10 per cent excluding references, figure and tables, thereby replicating criteria which many journals require for papers submitted to them.

ACTIVITY 8.3

Why would being able to understand and undertake research be beneficial to a doctor throughout their career? Try to list three reasons for doctors undertaking a mainly academic career and doctors taking a mainly non-academic career. Why are these skills important for all doctors to have? Have you undertaken any research projects already which could be included on your CV?

Intercalated degrees

Many UK institutions offer intercalated degrees. This is an extra year of study where you can gain an additional degree (e.g. BSc, BA, MSc or BMedSci). These usually have a strong research component to them and will complement and enhance the skills you will develop in SSCs. Almost a third of students will intercalate and for a small number of medical schools, such as Imperial College, London and Oxford and Cambridge Universities, they are now compulsory. Certainly, for students planning an academic career or for those who will become involved in research as doctors intercalated degrees can be useful, indeed they can be invaluable in giving the skills needed for a career in academic medicine.

Again, an intercalated degree can look impressive on a CV. Not only can it help doctors applying for consultant jobs, particularly in the more popular specialties, but an intercalated degree can gain points when students apply for foundation posts (see Chapter 11). It does mean, however, that students who do intercalate will graduate a year later than their peers so will incur higher loans and fees and will lose one year of earnings working as a doctor.

Some students feel that intercalated degrees are only for 'high achievers', but it's worth remembering that as you have already become a medical student you are already a high achiever. Intercalated degrees can also be used to broaden your knowledge base. For example, a student who is thinking that they may wish to be a surgeon may chose to intercalate in anatomy to improve anatomical knowledge.

What's the evidence?

- *Graduates with intercalated degrees gain higher marks in subsequent medical school exams.*
- *They are more likely to have papers published in peer reviewed journals and attract research grants.*
- *They may have an increased ability to evaluate research and understand methodological principles.*

(Cleland et al., 2009)

ACTIVITY 8.4

Many students say they don't have enough information about taking an intercalated degree. Next time you get the opportunity, talk to one of your teachers, your personal tutor, careers advisor, a junior doctor or an older student about intercalating.

Electives

All universities offer a final part of SSC – an elective – and these were offered before curricula in the UK embraced the recommendations of either edition of *Tomorrow's Doctors* so are the 'original' SSCs. Typically, these electives will last between 6 and 12 weeks, but this varies from medical school to medical school.

What's the evidence?

The BMA, MDU, MPS, MDUSS, the NHS (in Medical Careers) all have good information about electives, as well as *Projects Abroad: The Medic's Guide to Work and Electives Around the World* by Mark Wilson (2004), which is a good starting point to finding out about undertaking an elective outside the UK.

The goals of electives are to broaden students' undergraduate education through:

- providing the opportunity to explore new disciplines or old disciplines in greater detail;
- encouraging students to spend time learning outside the region where they are at medical school, including overseas attachments;
- giving students an opportunity to undertake an original research project.

Electives can also be used as an opportunity to learn about yourself and visit a part of the world you may never have considered visiting. Many students make the effort to go abroad during their electives and this can broaden clinical experiences particularly in countries which have a less developed health service than the UK. Therefore, electives can be good at developing transferable skills and showing future employers you can use your initiative Also, given the fact you will be in one place for a few weeks there is often the chance to undertake an audit or research project in areas which may not be offered at the university you are studying at. Again, gaining new experiences on an elective can also enhance a CV and be used to help meet person specifications when applying for jobs. Going to a developing country may allow you to do relief work and have hands-on experience with patients, whereas undertaking an elective in a developed country may allow you access to equipment you wouldn't see in the NHS.

Medical schools have lists of former places that students have been to and will be made available to you. Your head of year, student representative or personal tutor should know how to access this list if it isn't already available to you on your medical school website. They may know an organisation you can gain sponsorship from. In some developing countries you may be working providing aid which may attract sponsorship from charities or local businesses. Alternatively, you may find you are attracted to a specific specialty and wish to explore that, possibly with a view to a potential career path. If this is the case, a consultant or professor in your medical school should have contacts of names in the field.

As a student you will be a member of a medical union. Unions such as the Medical Protection Society (MPS) or Medical Defence Union (MDU) run electives. For example, according to the MDU website they have database of over 4000 hospitals and medical schools in more than 110 countries, an extensive funding database, student reports and forums, plus electives with a difference, including ones with Pfizer, the Prison Health Service, NASA and more. They also offer advice on flights and accommodation.

There are a few things to be aware of though. If you go to a remote place it may be difficult to keep in touch with family and friends. Going to a country with limited medicines and where many people do not speak your language can be daunting, although many students who go far afield often arrange electives with friends. You will need to consider where you will stay, travel insurance and you will need injections or visas to take an elective in certain countries. You also have to remember to stick within the guidelines you would be under if you were on any clinical attachments at home. You will be expected to maintain the same standards of professionalism as on any other undergraduate placement (see Chapter 3) and it is not unknown for students to be reported for unprofessional behaviour while on electives.

You must not behave as if or lead people to believe that you are a qualified doctor. You must work within the standards laid down by the GMC in *Tomorrow's Doctors* and *Good Medical Practice*. If you are travelling to a remote area it would be worth researching how the health system works in that country before you travel.

ACTIVITY 8.5

Ideally, where would you like to take an undergraduate medical elective? What advantages and disadvantages are there to travelling abroad for your elective? If you were to go abroad how would you finance the trip? Put 'medical electives' into Google and see how many websites it shows you. Look through the websites and see which of the electives offered would interest you.

Scenario three

Gemma undertook a laboratory-based SSC in her first year at medical school and really enjoyed the atmosphere of the laboratory and the excitement of experiments and looking through microscopes. She followed this up by undertaking a microbiology elective at a US university where she really enjoyed herself and felt she fitted in well in the team. Between her fourth and final year she undertook an intercalated degree in immunology. The references she got from the doctors who supervised her on her SSC and intercalated degree were a big help when she applied for a microbiology training post after her foundation training, which also enabled her to undertake an MSc while working as a microbiology trainee.

What's the evidence?

SSCs have now become an essential element of undergraduate medical curricula in the UK and could arguably be considered their most innovative aspect. The skills gained in SSCs both compliment the core curriculum and contribute to the attainment of the overall GMC learning outcomes. SSCs provide the student with an opportunity to learn a wide range of professional and lifelong learning skills to build upon during their professional careers and to maintain good medical practice. They often generate stimulating and challenging experiences for both students and staff.

(Riley, 2009)

Chapter summary

- SSCs can give invaluable experience which will help you develop skills as a doctor after you have graduated, such as developing research and evaluation skills including literature searching skills which are vital to all doctors.

- There are a wide variety of SSCs (including electives and intercalated degrees) which will allow you to choose an area of medicine or a medicine related subject that interests you and explore it in more depth.

- SSCs can help improve your CV, which may make you more attractive to employers when applying for jobs in your postgraduate career.

GOING FURTHER

- Murdoch-Eaton, D, Ellershaw, J, Garden, A, Newble, D, Perry, M, Robinson, L, Smith, J, Stark, P and Whittle, S (2004) Student-selected components in the undergraduate medical curriculum: a multi-institutional consensus on purpose. *Medical Teacher*, 26: 33–38.
  This article gives an excellent in-depth overview of the skills students can learn on SSCs.

- Murphy, J, De Senaviratne, R, Remers, O and Davis, M (2009) Student selected components: student-designed modules are associated with closer alignment of planned and learned outcomes. *Medical Teacher*, 31: 489–483.

- Riley, S (2009) Student Selected Components (SSCs): AMEE Guide number 46. *Medical Teacher*, 31: 885–894.
  This article and the one above are available on the internet. Again, they clearly show that there are common goals with all SSCs in UK universities.

- Wai-Ching Leung (2001) Is studying for an intercalated degree a wise career move? *StudentBMJ*, 09: 399–444. http://archive.student.bmj.com/issues/01/11/careers/418.php (accessed February 2011).
  This article gives you further information on the advantages and disadvantages of taking an intercalated degree.

- Wilson, M (2004) *The Medic's Guide to Work and Electives around the World.* London: Arnold.
  This book gives a useful guide to medical electives.

- World Federation for Medical Education (2003) *Basic Medical Education: WFME Global Standards for Quality Improvement.* www.wfme.org (accessed February 2011).
  This document gives an international overview to SSCs.

chapter 9

Peer Feedback on the Professional Behaviours of Medical Students

Jayne Garner

Achieving your medical degree

This chapter will help you begin to meet the following requirements of *Tomorrow's Doctors* (GMC, 2009a):

Outcomes 3 – The doctor as a professional

21. Reflect, learn and teach others.

(c) Continually and systematically reflect on practice and whenever necessary, translate that reflection into action, using improvement techniques and audit appropriately – for example, by critically appraising the prescribing of others.
(e) Recognise own personal and professional limits and seek help from colleagues and supervisors when necessary.
(f) Function effectively as a mentor and teacher including contributing to the appraisal, assessment and review of colleagues, giving effective feedback, and taking advantage of opportunities to develop these skills.

It will also introduce you to the following academic standards as set out in the GMC's guidance *Medical Students: Professional Values and Fitness to Practise* (GMC, 2009b):

(21) Doctors and students must be willing to contribute to the teaching, training, appraising and assessing of students and colleagues. They are also expected to be honest and objective when appraising or assessing the performance of others, in order to ensure students and colleagues are maintaining a satisfactory standard of practice
(22c) In order to demonstrate that they are fit to practise, students should be willing to contribute to the education of other students.

Chapter overview

Giving and receiving feedback is part of the lifelong learning and professional development expected of doctors. As an undergraduate medical student, you will give objective and honest feedback on the performance and behaviour of your colleagues. You are also expected to welcome such feedback on your own practice. This is part of being a professional and will help you reflect on your own skills and those of others. Giving and receiving feedback is a valuable learning opportunity, and you are encouraged to be constructive and understanding of such feedback as part of your development.

After reading this chapter you will be able to:

- distinguish what is meant by peer feedback and professional behaviours;
- appreciate the importance of peer feedback to your personal reflection and development;
- appreciate how to give and receive peer feedback on professional behaviours;
- be able to provide specific, evidence-based feedback.

Introduction

The General Medical Council (GMC) and the Medical Schools Council (MSC) recently updated their publication *Medical Students: Professional Behaviour and Fitness to Practise*, which highlights the importance of the professional behaviour of undergraduate medical students:

> *Medical students have certain privileges and responsibilities different from those of other students. Because of this, different standards of professional behaviour are expected of them. Medical schools are responsible for ensuring that medical students have opportunities to learn and practise the standards expected of them.*
>
> (GMC, 2009b, page 4)

The GMC also outline their expectations with regard to giving and receiving feedback in *Tomorrow's Doctors* (GMC, 2009a). This agenda is echoed in the GMC's emphasis on lifelong learning and the ability to reflect on and learn about your own practice:

> *Students must receive regular information about their development and progress. This should include feedback on both formative and summative assessments. . . . All doctors, other health and social care workers, patients and carers who come into contact with the student should have an opportunity to provide constructive feedback about their performance. Feedback about performance in assessments helps to identify strengths and weaknesses, both in students and in the curriculum, and this allows changes to be made.*
>
> (GMC, 2009a, paragraph 111)

The GMC also publishes guidance entitled *Good Medical Practice: Duties of a Doctor*, which highlights how it expects doctors to behave:

You are personally accountable for your professional practice and must always be prepared to justify your decisions and actions.

(GMC, 2006)

As part of your undergraduate medical curriculum, you will be encouraged to reflect on your experiences during small group sessions such as clinical or communication skills, anatomy classes or on clinical placements. This might be part of a formal evaluation process or a portfolio of evidence you are required to keep in order to demonstrate what you have learned. You may also have the opportunity to observe and comment on different aspects of your peers' practice including their contribution to team work, how they help other students, their professional behaviour and their performance when dealing with patients on clinical attachments.

This may be termed as peer feedback, peer appraisal, peer assessment, peer evaluation or peer nomination. For the purpose of this chapter, we will use the term 'peer feedback' as giving and receiving feedback is the key focus here. Opportunities for feedback will help you to reflect on your own development and will help make you a better, more self-aware doctor. The GMC specifies that:

You must provide only honest, justifiable and accurate comments when giving references for, or writing reports about, colleagues. When providing references you must do so promptly and include all information that is relevant to your colleague's competence, performance or conduct.

(GMC, 2010, paragraph 19)

It is important to emphasise that peer feedback can highlight your good points which are not recognised in the formal curriculum; for example, you might draw great diagrams that your peers find helpful or be excellent at listening to other people's points of view or ideas. This feedback is a useful way to identify your strong points, as well as the areas you can improve on. When we have conducted peer feedback in Liverpool, the vast majority of comments are very positive, as you will see later in this chapter.

But it must be acknowledged that giving negative constructive feedback – especially if it is face to face and you are accountable for your comments – can be daunting at first. If you have not had the opportunity to give such feedback to a colleague or peer before, it can be an uncomfortable experience and you may worry about offending or upsetting people. It is hoped that we can help you understand why this is a necessary part of your career as a doctor, and a necessary part of your role according to the GMC.

You must be honest and objective when appraising or assessing the performance of colleagues, including locums and students. Patients will be put at risk if you describe as competent someone who has not reached or maintained a satisfactory standard of practice.

(GMC, 2010, paragraph 18)

The skill of giving and receiving peer feedback links to the personal reflection elements of this book featured in the chapters on assessment (see Chapter 5) and communication (see Chapter 6).

What is meant by professional behaviour?

One clear definition of professional behaviour is provided by Arnold and Stern (2006), who state:

> *Professionalism is demonstrated through a foundation of clinical competence, commu-*
> *nication skills and ethical and legal understanding, upon which is built the aspiration*
> *to and wise application of the principles of professionalism: excellence, humanism,*
> *accountability and altruism.*

Key terms associated with professional behaviours are: honesty, empathy, compassion and respect for patients and colleagues. As a medical student you are expected to treat other people politely and considerately, including your peers. You should protect confidential information, and the dignity and privacy of your patients at all times. Definitions of professional behaviours are discussed in more depth as part of Chapter 3.

ACTIVITY 9.1 PEER FEEDBACK

Think about different ways you can give peer feedback, either formally or infor-mally. Rank the examples you can think of in terms of how useful you think they are. Discuss these with your peers; say why you think some of the feedback is more useful than others and why this is.

Why should I feed back on my peers' professional behaviour?

While you are a student, you are also in a good position to observe the actions and behaviour of your peers. You spend time with them in different settings – in small learning groups, taking on joint research projects, on clinical placements or other sport and social societies or clubs. You interact with your peers on a regular basis, and even though it might be subconscious, you observe their actions and words.

So you will know who is well prepared, who spends a lot of time in the library, who is most likely to volunteer to lead or chair a project. You will also know who is likely to be late, not turn up at all or will be in the pub! You know a lot about your peers probably without even realising it!

This is important. Papadakis *et al.* (2005) investigated the association between disciplinary action against practising physicians in the United States and prior unprofessional behaviour in medical school. They found that disciplinary action by a medical board was strongly associated with prior unprofessional behaviour in medi-cal school. So a link has been established between poor behaviour at medical school and subsequent disciplinary action against qualified doctors. What current medical educators wish to do is identify and support students who might be struggling or displaying unprofessional behaviour early in their careers.

One way to do this informally is by peer feedback: if this kind of unprofessional behaviour can be identified and raised by peers, it will be easier to address informally without becoming a fitness to practise issue or anything more serious.

The GMC expect you as a doctor to put the safety of your patients first. Whether you are a medical student or a fully qualified doctor, you have a responsibility to report and explain any concerns you have regarding the practice of colleagues.

> *You must protect patients from risk of harm posed by another colleague's conduct, performance or health. The safety of patients must come first at all times. If you have concerns that a colleague may not be fit to practise, you must take appropriate steps without delay, so that the concerns are investigated and patients protected where necessary. This means you must give an honest explanation of your concerns to an appropriate person from your employing or contracting body and follow their procedures.*
>
> (GMC, 2010, paragraph 43)

Furthermore, giving and receiving feedback is part of day-to-day life in the NHS. As a doctor you will have annual 360-degree feedback sessions to reflect on your lifelong learning and identify any training or support needs you may have. Part of a doctor's revalidation process similarly involves reflecting on feed back from different sources. So the more opportunity you have to give and receive feedback as an undergraduate medical student, the better you will be at it when you are a qualified doctor.

Scenario one

Amy and Josh started the MBChB course together, registering at the same session. They began a relationship during fresher's week, but Amy had a boyfriend back home in Sheffield and decided to finish things with Josh after a few weeks. Josh was very upset about this, and told other people on the course that she treated him badly. In the second semester, Josh was asked to feed back anonymously on Amy's professional behaviour as part of a communication skills exercise. Josh is still upset about his break up with Amy. Josh debates:

- speaking to the course tutor and asking to be re-assigned another student to feed back about;
- trying to complete an objective feedback of Amy's communication skills concentrating only on the criteria specified as part of the exercise;
- using the opportunity to criticise everything about Amy's communication skills because it's anonymous and it will upset her.

Josh decides to speak to the course tutor about feeding back on another student so he can complete the exercise fairly.

Why should I listen to my peers when tutors are the experts?

You might be sceptical about the opinions of your peers when you know they are at the same level as you and still learning. Yet, they may have noted small things that might be helpful for you to know; for example, you might not realise you have a tendency to dominate discussion and do not always give other people in the group a chance to speak, or you might have a really good knowledge of anatomy that people want you to speak more about. Peer feedback is a good way to learn about how you come across to other people and improve your communications skills (see also Chapter 6).

Also, your peers are an ideal source of observation and comment. It is also worth mentioning that peer feedback need not be limited to small group evaluation requirements or ward round reflections. You will have the opportunity to meet older students on the course through mentoring or social groups and societies. These students are an excellent source of feedback, as they have experienced first hand what stage of the course you are at, and what kind of feedback will be helpful to you. Don't be afraid to ask for feedback, most students are happy to be asked.

If you are unsure about asking for or giving feedback then your personal or clinical skills tutor will be able to offer you guidance. They are likely to have experience of peer or colleague feedback, so should be able to provide you with examples or to signpost where you can find similar information.

What if I upset a peer with constructive criticism, or they upset me?

It is more than likely you will receive constructive criticism at some stage of your education or career (you may even have already had this). The important thing to remember is that you can learn from feedback – it is part of your personal development. In truth it can be disheartening to receive some negative comments, but how you react and use this information says a lot about your professional persona.

You could get defensive and try to point out a flaw in the feedback you have received. But this probably would not make you look terribly mature or considered, especially if it is face to face. If you feel some feedback you have received is genuinely unfair or wrong then you should discuss it with a tutor, mentor or whoever you feel comfortable with. With some objective reflection you might see it differently.

It is also important to remember when you are giving feedback to a peer to be as concise as possible and provide evidence for your comments, especially if the feedback is given anonymously. This will make it easier for the recipient to understand and hopefully avoid any confusion or misunderstandings. You should always be prepared to justify your peer feedback; you are accountable for your comments, just as your peers are accountable for theirs.

Finally, do not take any constructive criticism personally as this is almost certainly not how it was meant. Try and be objective about it and appreciate it was meant to be helpful for your learning and reflection.

Scenario two

Following a ward round, Helen and Rob were asked by the consultant they were on placement with to present some feedback on each other's interaction with the patients they have seen. Rob wasn't paying attention because he had a late night, and he was tired, but he wants to impress the consultant. Rob debated:

- making up something vague about Helen's interaction with the patients and hoping they'd move along to something else;
- admitting he hadn't been fully observing Helen's interaction and asking if they can do this next time with some agreed criteria before they start;
- talking about his own interaction with patients, saying that if Helen behaved more like him, she would do much better in the future.

Rob decides to admit he hadn't been observing Helen's interaction and suggests they do the exercise next time.

Step by step feedback

Some of the skills you will need to objectively feed back upon the behaviour of your peers will be:

- observation – watching how people interact and remembering what they do and say;

- making notes of these observations and being prepared to phrase them in a useful and constructive way, using accessible language;

- remembering to give feedback at an appropriate agreed time and place – in front of a patient or consultant might not be suitable;

- being professional and limiting your comments to what is relevant, not your own interpretation of what should have been said or done.

ACTIVITY 9.2 PEER FEEDBACK

Try doing your own feedback with your student colleagues; you can do this either face to face, over a coffee, for example, or anonymously. You can pick an exercise such as a presentation or a small group project to feed back on. Practise how you phrase and present your feedback; try to anticipate how it will be received and what your peers will learn from it. Did you have any situations when you were at school or maybe involved in a sports team that you can draw on when you receive or give feedback? Try to make your feedback as detailed and constructive as possible.

Scenario three

Mina was asked to give peer feedback on one of her colleagues face to face. She was intimidated by the peer colleague, who she considered to be very loud, overly confident and 'leery' with the girls in their group. Mina debates:

- talking to a tutor about how she feels towards this colleague, and asking for support when she is giving feedback;
- bracing herself and telling the peer colleague why he intimidates her, and that some girls in the group might find his behaviour inappropriate;
- making an unnecessary appointment with the dentist so she misses the feedback session and doesn't have to give the peer feedback at all.

Mina decides to give the peer feedback face to face and explain fully why she finds her colleague intimidating and difficult, and discuss this issue with him.

What's the evidence?

- Peer assessment is an important part of developing professionalism in a medical curriculum (Elliott et al., 2009).
- Peer feedback and assessment can enhance students' performance at medical school (Schonrock-Adema et al., 2007).
- Peer feedback can help students develop communication skills (Perrera et al., 2010).

Case studies of peer feedback

In Liverpool we used an electronic-based anonymous comment system with second- and first-year students to provide them with experience of giving and receiving peer feedback on professional behaviours for their own personal reflection. Students were sent an e-mail asking them for feedback on two peers in their problem-based learning group. This was a formative exercise – it did not involve any scores or grades. The guidance we provided to students described the value of peer feedback and how it was to be undertaken:

- This is a valuable opportunity for you to learn about yourself and others – we expect you to be professional, and not abuse the peer feedback system with regard to personal grudges.

- The more detail you provide in a peer feedback the better – this is your chance to practise giving feedback and phrasing it appropriately.

- Please do not get offended by any constructive criticism – this is meant to help you learn about yourself, and aid reflection on your own behaviours.

- Please keep the feedback positive – if you are making a constructive comment back this up with evidence of what made you submit it – overall we want peer feedback to be positive with no negative, unnecessary, hurtful or offensive feedback.

- Remember this is part of your development as a medical professional and we hope you will treat it as such!

Students e-mailed comments back to the administrator, which were then sent onto the students to guarantee anonymity. Six examples of the peer feedback received from first-year students at the University of Liverpool are provided here:

1. [Name] is punctual to all PBL sessions and always arrives on time. She is happy to listen to others and is always enthusiastic during sessions. [Name] is very good at communicating herself clearly and whatever point she has she always explains in good depth. When [name] chaired a session, she took on the leadership role well and moved us along effectively. A minor area of improvement would be to maybe contribute more to discussions through drawing on the board more and taking on a more active role within the group. Overall, [name] is a friendly, patient person who many others would be happy to work with again.

2. I am sure he has things to bring to the table, but he doesn't bring them. I don't know what issues are holding him down, but whatever they are, they need to be resolved. And I say this in not in a nasty way, but in order for him to move forward.

3. [Name] is a really valuable member of the PBL group; she always contributes and explains tricky concepts well to everyone. From her performance you can tell that she works a lot and tries her best to cover all the learning objectives. She has a very nice manner about her and can correct people without sounding conde-scending or interruptive. I can't see any real areas for improvement apart from learning things a bit more to make it easier to explain things sometimes and getting up to draw things on the board more.

4. [Name] is a difficult individual to appraise, because I do not know if he does his work but does not speak, or if he does not do his work. I feel that he isolates himself from the rest of the group during the PBL sessions. He will participate if asked to, but never voluntarily. I feel that he is always distant; either uninterested or preoccupied, I do not know.

5. [Name]'s attendance to PBL sessions is unflawed and he is always well prepared and manages to recall a lot of information, particularly anatomy. He is a self con-fessed 'shy guy' but he has certainly come out of his shell since our first session.

It's necessary to say that perhaps [name] should pay attention when the girls in the group are talking as this is when he becomes slightly restless and engages in conversation about other things, generally football.

6. Very good student. Always well prepared and definitely does the work for each of the sessions. She likes to participate openly and willingly.

Think about how useful these examples of feedback are, and how such comments would help your own reflection and personal learning and how they could be applied to the teaching sessions at your medical school and in your curriculum.

Chapter summary

In this chapter you have found out:

- why peer feedback is important to the GMC and personal learning;

- what issues you might have in relation to peer feedback;

- consideration when giving and receiving peer feedback;

- examples of peer feedback.

GOING FURTHER

- Guidance from the GMC and the MSC on professional behaviour and fitness to practise for undergraduate medical students details what is expected of you as a medical student, and your responsibilities to others: www.gmc-uk.org/education/undergraduate/professional_behaviour.asp.

- Further guidance from the GMC outlines what they expect from doctors registered with them, and how they can best work with colleagues, patients and their families or carers: www.gmc-uk.org/guidance/good_medical_practice/duties_of_a_doctor.asp.

chapter 10

Clinical Placements

Andrew Bowhay

Achieving your medical degree

This chapter will help you to begin to meet the following requirements of *Tomorrow's Doctors* (GMC, 2009a):

Outcomes 2 – The doctor as a practitioner

13. The graduate will be able to carry out a consultation with a patient.

    (a) Take and record a patient's medical history, including family and social history, talking to relatives or other carers where appropriate.
    (b) Elicit patients' questions, their understanding of their condition and treatment options, and their views, concerns, values and preferences.
    (c) Perform a full physical examination.
    (d) Perform a mental-state examination.
    (e) Assess a patient's capacity to make a particular decision in accordance with legal requirements and the GMC's guidance (in Consent: Patients and doctors making decisions together).
    (f) Determine the extent to which patients want to be involved in decision-making about their care and treatment.
    (g) Provide explanation, advice, reassurance and support.

14. Diagnose and manage clinical presentations.

    (a) Interpret findings from the history, physical examination and mental-state examination, appreciating the importance of clinical, psychological, spiritual, religious, social and cultural factors.
    (b) Make an initial assessment of a patient's problems and a differential diagnosis. Understand the processes by which doctors make and test a differential diagnosis.
    (c) Formulate a plan of investigation in partnership with the patient, obtaining informed consent as an essential part of this process.
    (d) Interpret the results of investigations, including growth charts, x-rays and the results of the diagnostic procedures in Appendix 1.
    (e) Synthesise a full assessment of the patient's problems and define the likely diagnosis or diagnoses.
    (f) Make clinical judgments and decisions, based on the available evidence, in

conjunction with colleagues and as appropriate for the graduate's level of training and experience. This may include situations of uncertainty.

(g) Formulate a plan for treatment, management and discharge, according to established principles and best evidence, in partnership with the patient, their carers, and other health professionals as appropriate. Respond to patients' concerns and preferences, obtain informed consent, and respect the rights of patients to reach decisions with their doctor about their treatment and care and to refuse or limit treatment.

(h) Support patients in caring for themselves.

(i) Identify the signs that suggest children or other vulnerable people may be suffering from abuse or neglect and know what action to take to safeguard their welfare.

(j) Contribute to the care of patients and their families at the end of life, including management of symptoms, practical issues of law and certification, and effective communication and team working.

Chapter overview

This chapter will help you to know what learning opportunities are available in the clinical environment and how best to make the most of these opportunities.

Learning directly from patients is one of the most important parts of medical training and is something that continues from the first day you meet a patient to the final day of a your career as a doctor. It is therefore important that you take advantage of all the opportunities that arise in your undergraduate training to interact with patients and trainers in the clinical environment.

After reading this chapter you will be able to:

- know what training in the clinical environment will be available to enhance your learning about patients and their diseases and treatments;
- understand why training in the clinical environment is such an important part of the medical school curriculum;
- understand why reflecting on your learning is an important aspect of the professional life of a student as well as a doctor.

Learning in the clinical environment

Learning directly from patients is something that the General Medical Council (GMC) expects every medical undergraduate curriculum to undertake. In its document *Tomorrow's Doctors* (GMC, 2009a), the GMC states that the curricula:

will include practical experience of working with patients throughout all years, increasing in duration and responsibility so that graduates are prepared for their responsibilities as provisionally registered doctors. It will provide enough structured clinical placements to enable students to demonstrate the 'outcomes for graduates' across a range of clinical specialties, including at least one Student Assistantship period.

(GMC, 2009a, paragraph 48)

The clinical environment that supports this practical experience will be in a variety of settings which will include hospital inpatient and outpatient departments but also, increasingly, will be in the community such as in general practice surgeries. Each of these settings has their own distinct challenges, but it is during these placements that you will learn what it means to be a real doctor. Some of the skills that you will learn in the clinical skills classroom, such as history taking, physical examining, practical procedures, communication and professionalism, will now take on a new meaning and relevance and the medical knowledge that you have learnt in the lecture theatre can also be applied to patient care; this linking of apparently academic facts to the real life patient helps to embed and make relevant this knowledge and drive self-directed learning.

The first interactions with patients, however, can be stressful for students as you may feel unprepared for clinical learning because the environment can appear to be initially intimidating, particularly if there has been a lack of guidance from the medical school. The clinical environment, whether a GP's surgery or a hospital ward, will be very different from the usual undergraduate milieu, and the necessity to dress in a standard manner and to think about personal appearance is very different from the casual dress codes of non-medical students. In addition you will have to interact with medical staff and patients and to perform clinical tasks which may not yet be routine (Shacklady *et al.*, 2009).

Case study: Meet your first patient

Riona is a medical student preparing to go on her first clinical attachment at a hospital. The hospital has an undergraduate co-ordinator who has arranged to meet all the new students on the first morning to give them an induction talk and arrange identification (ID) badges. The co-ordinator talked about dress code as well as telling the students that there were a few wards they could not go to on their own, such as the intensive care unit (ICU). However, they were also told that they could go onto the ICU if that was part of the consultant's or registrar's ward round.

The undergraduate co-ordinator had already allocated Riona and another student to meet Dr Jones, who is a specialist registrar in medicine, on Ward Q at 13.30 hours so that they would have their first experience of working on a ward and also have the opportunity to take a history and examine a patient for the first time. Riona and her colleague had already done this in the clinical skills laboratory, but being on a ward did seem different. She noted more background noise, particularly from televisions, and more hustle and bustle as nurses attended patients. Dr Jones introduces them to the nurse in charge of the ward and told them what types of patient illnesses were treated and investigated on Ward Q.

They were then introduced to Mrs Smith who had been admitted for investigations and Riona asked if she would mind her taking a history; her colleague examined Mrs Smith. Once they had finished they went back to Dr Jones who asked them to tell her what they had found and also give some possible diagnoses and what investigations would help confirm these.

Riona and her colleague talked afterwards about how they felt they had managed, what they had done well and what could be improved for next time. Riona found talking to her colleague really useful as they both realised that they had both been nervous seeing their first patient.

What do I need to know before I meet my first patient?

What should I wear?

Medical students are not expected to wear the equivalent of a three-piece suit; however, you should also not be dressed as if you are about to go out on a Saturday night! 'Smart casual' would seem to fit expectations but this should be also guided by local policies. For instance, most hospitals now have infection control policies and these may say that white coats should not be worn; ties may or may not be worn but if worn must be tucked into the shirt so they do not dangle; long hair must be tied back; arms should be bare below the elbow with rings being restricted to a single metal band; any chains worn must not be visible; earrings should be studs with no dangling earrings; fingernails should be short with no false nails as these can become detached and also prevent effective handwashing; and makeup should be in keeping with promoting a professional image.

It should also be remembered that medicine does require a lot of bending over or bending down in front of patients and therefore for female students skirts and blouses in particular should be appropriate to allow you to do that without revealing more than you would want to reveal.

How do I get access to the clinical areas and how will I be identified?

The medical school will arrange an ID badge for you, but each hospital may require their own ID badge, particularly where the badge also acts as a means for entering clinical areas that are secured with magnetic security locks. These ID badges may be called 'swipe cards' as they have to be swiped through or over a detector to unlock the appropriate door. The badge will have a photo of you, your name and status and it will need to be visible at all times. It is important, therefore, that your face is not covered so that you can be easily identified.

In the operating theatre you will also be asked to identify yourself at the start of the operating list, as do all staff, as part of the routine World Health Organization (WHO) checklist.

Can I go and see any patient?

You should ask the person in charge of the ward or clinic or the most senior doctor whether you can go and see a patient. You need to make sure the patient is well enough and capable of being interviewed or examined. A doctor on the ward may be able to tell you which patients have good symptoms and signs; however you do need to make sure the patient consents to being seen by you. You should introduce yourself to the patient and there is some evidence that patients prefer the term 'student doctor' rather than 'medical student' (Chipp *et al.*, 2004). It is important that you (or any doctor for that matter) do not leave yourself in situations where you are completely alone with a patient and where there are no chaperones, so it is often better to interview patients in pairs.

What equipment do I require to see patients?

If you are going to take a history and examine a patient you will need a pen and some paper to write down what you have found as there may be too much information to remember. Also, if you going to examine a patient you do need to have a stethoscope. Any other specialist equipment should be available in the clinical area.

How do students get into the operating theatre?

The operating theatres are quite different from the ward environment and are often accessed through changing rooms where everyone has to change into theatre suits, sometimes called 'scrubs'. The first time that you go into the operating theatre you should be shown round by a member of staff so you know where to go, what to wear and what you can or cannot touch (some of the trolleys will have sterile equipment on them and should not be touched unless wearing sterile gowns and gloves). The operating theatres do seem to be an even more alien environment than the wards and some of the procedures are very different and can make some people feel faint; hence it is advisable to have a good breakfast that morning!

> **ACTIVITY 10.1**
>
> Write a list of the places in the NHS where you think you will be able to learn directly from patients. Do you think that learning in the clinical environment will be different from the clinical skills laboratory and the lecture theatre? If different, why do you think that will be?

How will I be taught?

The clinical workplace is different from the lecture theatre or tutorial room in that the prime focus for the teacher in these situations is usually the students, but once you enter the clinical environment this relationship becomes tripartite, with the patient usually becoming the centre of attention. This does not mean that you will be neglected, but it is important for you to realise that there is now a three-way relationship between you, the trainer and the patient. In addition, while lectures may be planned well ahead of time and focus on a particular subject or disease, what is seen in the clinical environment will depend on which patients have been admitted to the hospital or arrive in the GP surgery, and hence your days may not seem as organised and will not follow a clearly defined timetable.

Nevertheless, the curriculum will have been planned and structured to give you experience across a range of specialties, rather than relying entirely upon this arising by chance. These specialties must include medicine, obstetrics and gynaecology, paediatrics, surgery, psychiatry and general practice (GMC, 2009a). Because patients now spend much less time in hospital than formerly it may be difficult to follow the natural history of a disease in one patient, but you will be able to piece together the natural history from a number of patient encounters, including encounters in the community.

The types of clinical encounters that you can expect will include:

- the consultant ward round;
- the working ward round with a doctor in training;
- a ward round or clinic with a specialist nurse;
- going to the operating theatre to watch surgical and anaesthetic procedures;
- attending outpatients with a consultant or a doctor in training;
- attending a GP surgery;
- attending multidisciplinary team meetings;
- going on home visits with a GP;
- going on visits to meet patients and their carers in their homes;
- taking a history and examining a patient on the ward, in the outpatient clinic or in a community setting.

ACTIVITY 10.2

Which of the clinical environments do you think will be the best place for you to learn?

Inpatient teaching, and hence learning, can be quite challenging for both the teacher and the student as it can seem a bit disorganised. This is because although the teacher may have set goals for the teaching, unanticipated events can frequently occur. Despite this, you should make sure you are always present at the allotted time and place.

The consultant ward round

The consultant ward round can be quite daunting for students as it will involve a variety of staff, often at different stages of training and with differing learning needs. Engaging all learners simultaneously can be difficult. You can learn a lot by watching how a senior doctor interacts with patients, particularly their history and examination techniques, clinical reasoning skills and professionalism. It is also true, however, that you may experience examples of poor practice which run counter to what you have learnt before; in other words, the doctor is not practising what they are teaching. It is important that you think about what you have seen and heard and decide whether you would wish to incorporate it into your practice. This difference in what is being taught and what is being seen and learnt by students is sometimes called the 'hidden curriculum' (Hafferty, 1998).

The working ward round

Working ward rounds with doctors in training do teach students how to manage the day-to-day tasks of working in a hospital. This is particularly important as the main outcome of undergraduate medical training is to ensure your preparedness for Foundation Year One (F1) training. Doctors in training will have also been students much more recently than consultants and should remember what it is like being a student on the ward; they will also have knowledge of all the patients under their care and should be able to guide you to patients with interesting clinical symptoms and signs. They are also likely to be about to take or have recently taken postgraduate examinations and hence their knowledge base is often very good.

Nurse specialists

Nurse specialists are nurses who have undertaken additional training and usually have a great wealth of experience in their area of practice. Unlike doctors in training, whose posts may be transitory in a particular department, nurse specialists tend to work in a department for many years and hence have a great understanding of the patients with chronic disease, particularly their social circumstances. In the community setting, a nurse specialist may be undertaking a large proportion of the screening programmes.

Attending the operating theatre

Attendance at operations is an important aspect of learning for medical students. While you may think that you do not wish to undertake surgery as a career, what happens in the operating theatre will impact on your working life at some point and having an understanding of what goes on will help you to answer questions from worried patients. In addition, various doctors, other than just surgeons, work in the operating theatres, and an exposure to their work may stimulate you to consider anaesthesia, for example, as a career option.

One aspect of learning that is very informative for students is seeing anatomy and procedures in three dimensions, and this does give a better understanding of the spatial relationship of the organs in the body for instance. Surgeons are very good sources on anatomical information and do like to ask students questions, particularly on anatomy. Anaesthetists have very good knowledge of physiology, pharmacology and how to manage the acutely ill patient.

Various procedures are undertaken in the operating theatre or in specialised units. Endoscopy procedures, for example, use an instrument, usually a fibreoptic telescope, to look inside hollow organs or body cavities. These are excellent ways of viewing disease; most endoscopes now have cameras with the images projected onto high-resolution screens so everyone can see what is happening.

Outpatient departments

Outpatient departments are usually very busy and as each patient encounter is often quite short there is often little time for elaborate teaching. With some organisation, however, it will possible for you to take a history and examine a patient which can then be presented succinctly to the doctor. New patients will usually come with referral letters which will have some details of the patient's problems. It is important during these encounters that you also think about differential diagnoses, further investigations and treatment plans so that you can feel part of the whole consultation process. The doctor in these circumstances may then act as your guide and facilitator rather than just an information provider. Patients will often come with multiple problems, some of which may have mixed organic and psychosocial origins, which must be addressed simultaneously; you need to be aware that the doctor cannot focus on one problem for teaching purposes.

GP surgeries

Placements in general practice are now an important part of medical training. The patient encounters in GP surgeries, like the hospital outpatient setting, are often quite short, but here the new patients can arrive with any problem ranging from psychiatric illnesses to problems that perhaps can only be treated by surgery. Therefore, it is important to let the patient tell you what is wrong with them. It may be that the problem they start to discuss is not what they are really worried about.

Learning how to take a history in a relatively short time is an important part of the learning experience and GPs are expert in this type of encounter. You will need to think about diagnoses and what further needs to be done because some conditions can be investigated and managed by the GP but others may need to be referred to a specialist in a hospital.

Attending multidisciplinary team meetings

Attending multidisciplinary team (MDT) meetings can be very instructive in how the many different professional groups work together to improve outcomes for patients. Many medical specialties will have MDTs to discuss complex patients who usually have chronic diseases, such as cystic fibrosis. The aim of these meetings is to explore all aspects of the patient's disease and incorporate the opinions from many different professional sources in one forum. The professional groups will include nurses, physiotherapists, occupational therapists, dieticians, social workers, etc.

Going on home visits with a GP

Going on home visits with a GP or going to meet patients and their carers in their homes as part of the medical course will enable you to see how patients live with disease and cope with illness in the community. The understanding of how patients live is an important aspect of the holistic care of the patient. You may also have the opportunity to go on domiciliary consultations with a consultant, which again gives the doctor the opportunity to review patients in their home surroundings and provides a better understanding of how their medical problems affect their lives.

ACTIVITY 10.3

Think about what differences there will be between your clinical training in the first and final years of your medical course. Why do you think they should be different? What do you think the difference is between being competent and expert at something?

Taking histories and examining patients

Taking histories and examining patients, whether in a hospital or a community setting, is an important part of learning and the more you undertake the more expert you will become in these skills. As with all skills, it is important that they are practised, but as part of experiential learning you will need to stand back and review what you have done; you will then need to learn from this review and apply what you have learnt when you next undertake a similar task or skill. Dennison and Kirk put it succinctly as 'Do, Review, Learn, Apply' (Dennison and Kirk, 1990). This cyclical learning process should be part of any doctor's learning and an inability to do this is a major cause of poor performance in doctors.

The later years of training

During the later years of medical school training, you should have the opportunity to become increasingly competent in your clinical skills and in planning patient care. You should therefore have a defined role in medical teams, be subject to considerations of patient safety, and this should become more central as your education continues (GMC, 2009a).

With this in mind, the GMC expects that in the final year of training you should have the opportunity to use your practical and clinical skills as a rehearsal for your eventual responsibilities as an F1 doctor. These opportunities must include making recommendations for the prescription of drugs, undertaking practical procedures such as taking blood and managing acutely ill patients under the supervision of a qualified doctor. The GMC states that this period of training should take the form of one or more student assistantships in which you, assisting a junior doctor and under supervision, will undertake most of the duties of an F1 doctor. The period of this assistantship will vary between medical schools, but can be of the order of seven weeks.

This period of training is perhaps the most important for the final-year student as it gives you the opportunity to experience what it is like to actually work as a doctor on the wards. While some medical schools have previously ensured that the assistantship you would undertake is the same post you would undertake at the start of your F1 posts, this is now not feasible with the national application process for the foundation programme. However, the GMC does recommend that wherever practicable, you should have a period working with the F1 who is in the post you will take up when you graduate.

This 'shadowing' period allows you to become familiar with the facilities available, the working environment, the working patterns as well as the opportunity to get to know your colleagues. It also provides an opportunity to develop working relationships with the clinical and educational supervisors you will work with in the future. It should consist of 'protected time' involving tasks that enable you to use your medical knowledge and expertise in a working environment, distinct from the general induction sessions provided for new employees and foundation programme trainees. The 'shadowing' period should normally last at least one week and take place as close to the point of employment as is feasible.

You should check in your final year of training if this 'shadowing' period is available for the F1 post you are allocated as this will vary between medical schools and hospitals.

Case study: Preparing for F1

Riona is now in her final year of medical school and is about to take her final examinations, but her last training placement is to shadow Dr Thomas Roberts who is the F1 doctor that Riona will take over from in August if she passes her examinations.

Riona meets Dr Roberts on Ward X3 at 09.00 and is introduced to Charge Nurse Andrew Collins who is the senior nurse in charge of the ward. Dr Roberts only works on one ward but he tells Riona that a number of different consultants have patients on the wards and so he has to go on quite a number of ward rounds during the week. That day there were going to be a number of routine admissions and Dr Roberts thought it would be useful for Riona to hone her history and examination skills by clerking in half of the patients. He would check the clerking and Riona should suggest relevant investigations, although he would order them as he had a password for the computer, but she could take the blood.

Just before 10.00 a consultant arrived with her SpR to see her patients. Dr Roberts and Riona followed the consultant and Dr Roberts gave the consultant a concise description of how the patients were and the results of any investigations. Riona was impressed that he seemed to know about the consultant's patients and wondered if she would be able to remember all this information in a few months' time.

During the ward round Riona noted that Dr Roberts was writing in the patients' notes and also noting down on a piece of paper what other investigations the consultant wanted undertaking. She realised that being an F1 doctor required good organisational and time management skills.

Chapter summary

This chapter has:

- explained why learning from patients is such an important part of training;

- indicated where and when patient interactions, and the subsequent learning and teaching, can take place;

- emphasised the importance of practice to improve skills;

- emphasised the importance of reflecting on practice as a means to improve.

GOING FURTHER

- Chipp, E, Stoneley, S and Cooper, K (2004) Clinical placements for medical students: factors affecting patients' involvement in medical education. *Medical Teacher*, 26(2): 114–119.
  This paper studied what factors affect a patient's willingness to be involved in medical education.

- Hutchinson, L (2003) Educational environment. *British Medical Journal*, 326(7393): 810–812.
  This paper is in the series 'ABC of learning and teaching', published by the BMJ in 2003 and discusses the engagement of learners particularly in the medical environment.

- Ramani, S and Leinster, S (2008) AMEE Guide no. 34: Teaching in the clinical environment. *Medical Teacher*, 30(4): 347–364.
  Although this article is aimed at clinical teachers it does help explain why clinical teaching is set up the way it is.

- Shacklady, J, Holmes, E, Mason, G, Davies, I and Dornan, T (2009) Maturity and medical students' ease of transition into the clinical environment. *Medical Teacher*, 31(7): 621–626.
  This article discusses the effects of moving into clinical training on medical students.

- Spencer, J (2003) Learning and teaching in the clinical environment. *British Medical Journal*, 326(7389): 591–594.
  This is another paper in the 'ABC of learning and teaching' series published by the BMJ in 2003 and focuses on learning in the clinical environment.

chapter 11

Career Planning and How to Build Your CV for a Career in Medicine
Christine Waddelove

Achieving your medical degree

This chapter will help you to begin to meet the following requirements of *Tomorrow's Doctors* (GMC, 2009a):

Outcomes 3 – The doctor as a professional

21. Reflect, learn and teach others.

(b) Establish the foundations for lifelong learning and continuing professional development, including a professional development portfolio containing reflections, achievements and learning needs.

Domain 6 – Support and development of students, teachers and the local faculty

125. Students will have access to career advice, and opportunities to explore different careers in medicine. Appropriate alternative qualification pathways will be available to those who decide to leave medicine.
134. Schools must have a careers guidance strategy. Generic resources should include an outline of career paths in medicine and the postgraduate specialties, as well as guidance on application forms and processes. Specific guidance should be provided for personalised career planning. The careers strategy should be developed and updated with the local postgraduate deanery.
135. A small number of students may discover that they have made a wrong career choice. Medical schools must make sure that these students, whose academic and non-academic performance is not in question, are able to gain an alternative degree or to transfer to another degree course.
136. Students who do not meet the necessary standards in terms of demonstrating appropriate knowledge, skills and behaviour should be advised of alternative careers to follow.

Chapter overview

It may seem a little premature to have a chapter on career planning and building your curriculum vitae (CV) when you have only just made a decision to study medicine. However, there are over 60 different specialties that you can enter as a doctor and many are very competitive. You need to be thinking not just about specialty areas that may be suitable but also, from an early stage, activities that you can undertake that will enhance your CV and help you to stand out from your peers when it comes to applying for jobs.

As a fundamental skill, all doctors should be able to manage their career and this is increasingly important because of the increasing variety of opportunities available and the constant changes occurring within the National Health Service (NHS). Being able to access information about different specialty areas as well as the ratio of applicants to places will be important. You will also need to develop a knowledge of yourself, your values, personality and skills that may suit a particular speciality area.

Your CV, which should be a detailed listing of your educational achievements, publications, presentations, professional activities and interests and work history, will help you to market yourself to future employers. It gives you the chance to 'sell' your skills and experiences and you will use it to emphasise your strong points – to make your application stand out. We encourage you to start keeping a record of your achievements both within and outside the curriculum and to build up your CV as you move through medical school.

In this chapter we will look at strategies to help you start planning for your future career and then look at some of the activities that you can undertake over the next few years to help you build your CV so that you can be successful in your chosen path. Although you do not necessarily always need to provide a CV for a job for some posts, no matter how you apply you will still need to be able to sell your academic, clinical and transferable skills to a future employer.

After reading this chapter you will be able to:

- understand what career planning is and how you might start to develop planning skills;
- become familiar with some activities and resources that may help you plan your career;
- consider how you may build your skills and your CV while at medical school.

Why career planning now?

It is useful to consider why you need to be thinking about career planning early in your medical undergraduate training. As we have noted already, there are over 60 different medical specialties which students can opt to train in and, in addition to which, there are various research and teaching options. Under the reforms of Modernising Medical Careers (MMC) (Department of Health, 2005), junior doctors now have to make a definitive choice about a career pathway much sooner than they have had to in the past, when many doctors used to work in standalone training posts, often over a number of years before deciding which specialty to train in (Watmough *et al.*, 2009, pages 51–59).

After graduation, medical students have to take a structured two-year training programme prior to embarking on specialist training called the Foundation Programme. There is also an academic route during Foundation which has a separate application process and is a route specially designed for students who may be interested in going into academic medicine. Medical graduates have to decide which route to take and apply for specialty posts less than 18 months after graduation, before they complete the Foundation Programme. There are also increasing numbers of medical graduates and increasing numbers of overseas doctors applying for posts, so competition has increased. Therefore it is important to develop career planning skills while at medical school. Figure 11.1 gives a structure chart for your career in medicine.

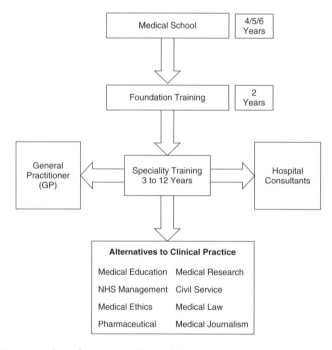

Figure 11.1 Structure chart for a career in medicine.

What's the evidence?

'Career management: an approach for medical schools, deaneries, royal colleges and trusts', put together by the Modernising Medical Careers (MMC) working group for career management in 2005 (Department of Health, 2005), states:

> an effective career management system must span the totality of undergraduate and postgraduate medical training, including recruitment of students into medical school.

Recommendation 17 in the Tooke Report (Tooke, 2008) emphasised the need for medical schools to play a greater role in providing careers information and advice:

> Career aspirations and choices should be informed by accurate data. Medical schools should play a greater role in careers advice.

How can you start to plan?

You actually started the process of career planning when you decided to take your medical degree and you will have a number of decisions to make during training which could influence your career choice, such as whether you go abroad for your elective placement, which student selected components (SSCs) to take or whether you should take an extra degree by intercalating. Even when you gain experience as a foundation doctor and specialist trainee you will still have career decisions to make, for example whether you want to work in a teaching hospital or district general hospital. Career planning is, therefore, a lifelong process; if you learn some of the skills while you are still at medical school the process will be made much easier throughout your career.

One of the first things you should do when you start medical school is to visit the careers' centre and see what services they offer. These may include helping you find voluntary work or vacation jobs, as well as useful workshops on topics such as how to write CVs. They will also normally have a careers adviser who is responsible for offering specific careers advice for medical students – so do check. To develop career planning skills it is necessary to go through a process, which includes becoming more self-aware, knowing how to explore and research options, being able to make a decision and then carrying the plan through.

Self-awareness

Self-assessment tools can be useful when considering your future career; remember that no set of results can tell you what specialty to choose, but they can help you in the process. Thinking about yourself is an extremely important aspect of career planning and there are various aspects to this, but consider undertaking exercises which will help you become more aware about your interests, skills, interests, motivations and personality.

Your career service should be able to provide you with suitable exercises. Otherwise, take a look at the www.medicalcareers.nhs.uk website. There is also an online resource which has been developed by the Open University called Sci59 Online. This has been designed to help medical students and junior doctors in training see how their skills, attitudes, preferences and aspirations map against specialties. Sci59 is free to British Medical Association (BMA) members (students can join the BMA) and may be available from your careers service.

You should also consider taking the Myers Briggs Type Indicator (MBTI). This can help you to understand your personality and temperament and although it is not directly linked to medicine, many students and junior doctors will find it very useful in helping them to become more self-aware. The inventory should be administered by a qualified MBTI practitioner.

ACTIVITY 11.1

When you are on attachments reflect upon your own qualities, what you are good at and enjoy and how this might suit your future speciality choice. Think about what you want to get out of work, what makes a job attractive to you (e.g. working as part of a team, being hospital based, working routine hours, working with a particular patient group, etc.).

Case study: Making choices

Helen was in her fourth year at medical school and had always thought that she would train to be a GP. During her attachment in a general practice she began to question whether this was the best specialty choice for her. She enjoyed working with the variety of patients but felt more comfortable when she did not have to become involved with the patients over a long period of time. She had a chat with the careers adviser for medicine, took a couple of online tests, including the Sci59, and together they looked at the results and talked about the specialties that could offer her the opportunity to see a variety of patients but to then refer them to other specialties.

During her fifth year she was able to do a placement in emergency medicine and thoroughly enjoyed the variety of patients she dealt with but also the fact that they were then either discharged or referred elsewhere. She hopes to take a rotation in this area in foundation training and is seriously now considering this specialty.

Career planning/exploration

You will be developing research skills in accessing and analysing information as part of your medical degree (see Chapter 8), but these also need to be applied to reviewing career opportunities.

This information can come from sources such as publications, people (from other doctors, careers advisers and your peers) or media.

ACTIVITY 11.2

There are lots of useful websites and activities that will help you learn more about the career structures within medicine.

- Information on the foundation programme: www.foundationprogramme.nhs. uk/pages/home.
- Information on specialty training: www.mmc.nhs.uk.
- Royal College websites – they often have specific sections on careers within that area.
- Attend careers fairs – the *British Medical Journal* usually hold an annual fair for medical students and junior doctors: http://careersfair.bmj.com/en/1/home. html or indeed your own medical school may hold fairs.
- Look at Centre for Workforce Intelligence (www.cfwi.org.uk/) for lots of statistics on different specialties and their competitiveness.

Decision making

You need to understand your personal decision-making style as you will be making decisions throughout your course (e.g. your choice of SSCs, whether to intercalate, where to live, how to spend your summer holidays). Few decisions are made completely on their own; there are often constraints on choice, or things which will carry additional weight in your selection criteria (e.g. cost of intercalation, location). It is important not to wait until you are at a major decision point (of course or job) but to develop an understanding of your personal style along the way.

You should understand how you usually tend to make decisions. For example do you:

- act spontaneously, deciding on a whim;
- only commit yourself after extensive information collation and research;
- choose things to please other people;
- opt out of decisions and let events control you?

If you are clear about this you can consciously choose to make decisions on a different basis in the future. See www.medicalcareers.nhs.uk/pdf.aspx?page=7025 for more information on how to make decisions.

Plan implementation

You will have to apply for electives or intercalation before you have to apply for your postgraduate posts and good applications are usually dependent on you drawing on the knowledge you have gained about yourself, the information you have gained about the opportunities, plus having insight into your normal decision-making style and factors influencing your choice.

You may even decide to plan for these applications by producing an action plan. Action planning can be very useful. Consider these three steps:

- Where am I now?

- Where do I want to be?

- How do I get there?

The ability to implement an action plan involves identifying steps needed for you to reach your goal.

The following information suggests ways in which medical undergraduates can start to develop their employability skills. Medical graduates are finding that having excellent academic and clinical skills may not quite be enough to secure the specialty of their choice. So in order to be successful in their application for the foundation programme or specialist training, applicants have to be able to show that they have the academic and clinical skills sought, and that in addition to these they have a range of transferable skills which will enable them to do the job effectively and to be a useful and effective employee from day one.

We can call this building your CV. There are plenty of opportunities to build your CV and help you stand out from your peers. Even the fun things you do like sports or music can develop your skills such as organisational or interpersonal skills. You may already have a CV and if you have you will need to continually update it if it is going to be of any real value and a true reflection of your experience and achievements.

ACTIVITY 11.3

If you don't have a CV then start considering compiling one (even if you are still three or four years away from making the transition from university to foundation training, you will still be applying for electives, vacation work, intercalation, bursaries and so forth and it is very likely that any such applications will ask for a CV). For examples of CVs see www.medicalcareers.nhs.uk/pdf.aspx?page=7641

Show it to someone such as a careers adviser, supervisor, tutor or doctor for comments.

Building your CV through external activities

Volunteering

Volunteering is an excellent way of gaining extra experience and developing your skills while also contributing to a community or a cause that is important to you. There are lots of different opportunities available, from helping young people in care to working with those with a disability or health problem. Through volunteering you can:

- improve key skills or add new skills and experience to your CV;
- make a difference to people's lives;
- make contacts so you can do some networking later;
- gain experience in the medical or social care field, or other areas where paid work experience is not usually available;
- show motivation and interest in specialty;
- get good references for your CV or application form;
- have fun!

Your careers department will usually have volunteer opportunities advertised.

Case study: Volunteer opportunities

Rob was in his first year of medical school when he received an e-mail from his careers service advertising a voluntary fair for students specifically from the health and medical departments. He went along and had a chat with a number of organisations who were looking for students to volunteer. He was particularly keen to work with people with mental health issues and from the fair he managed to gain a voluntary placement to work with teenagers suffering from mental health problems. He received mentor training and was then given the names of a couple of teenagers to help mentor. He enjoyed the work and met up with the young people on a regular basis to discuss their issues and offer practical support. The flexibility fitted in well with his timetable and he gained lots of transferable skills which will demonstrate that he is willing and able to take on new challenges and skills that will help make him stand out from his peers. He has now entered specialist training in psychiatry and believes that the experience and skills he developed during his voluntary work helped secure him the post.

Vacation work

There are a number of opportunities for students to work during their vacation periods ranging from serving in a bar or restaurant to teaching English overseas, working with children in holiday playgroups, or working as a health care assistant learning about their role and developing important skills at the same time. The opportunities are many; it is simply a case of taking the initiative and going for it! Whatever you want to do, start looking for vacation work early, especially if you want to work abroad. Many vacation work opportunities won't be advertised and many students find work as a result of speculative applications or by word-of-mouth. You may have to be a little creative in your search but do go to your careers service as a starting point.

Summer camp work

There are a number of organisations offering work for students in summer camps throughout the world. Well-recognised providers of such opportunities include British Universities North America Club (BUNAC) and Camp America. There are specialist summer camps which cater for children with, for example, disabilities and they may provide excellent skills development opportunities for you.

Societies

Getting involved in university or external societies, sporting teams and other such groups is a great way of gaining and demonstrating transferable skills to future employers. The university can offer you many societies from sports to charity work and usually the medical students will have their own societies, such as journal clubs, psychiatry society, surgical society, some of which should be of interest. If there isn't one that interests you, you could consider setting up a new society. For example, recently a mature students' society has been developed at a university by some students who felt a need for such a group to share issues that they felt are specific to them. In order to make the most of your participation you do need to be fully involved and if possible hold a specific and responsible role such as treasurer, chair, fundraiser or secretary but at least make a start by joining a society!

Student representative

There will be a number of opportunities throughout your medical degree to become a student representative. Their role is to ensure that your fellow students' views are listened to in the department. Similarly, when you start to have more clinical attachments you can become a rep who reports on the clinical attachments. Becoming a rep can give you excellent experience in presenting, negotiation and liaising with other medical students and academic and clinical staff.

Visit career fairs and events

These are highly valued by students and trainees who see them as a one-on-one opportunity to talk to specialists about careers and what it is really like to work in the specialty. The BMJ usually run at least one every year: http://careersfair.bmj.com/en/1/home.html

Building your CV through your medical degree and making yourself employable

Special study modules

Special study modules are compulsory periods of supervised study which are discussed in Chapter 8. You do not need to take every module with your future specialty in mind. Indeed, many of you will not have a clear idea of the eventual area you wish to specialise in. So what you do want to do is to keep a record of the skills that you have developed and if you can do at least one or two modules in an area of specific careers interest then great!

Electives

Details of electives can be found in Chapter 8 but do remember that your elective can be an exciting opportunity to explore areas of medicine in different cultures, specialties and social settings. This is an ideal opportunity to get involved in an area of medicine or to develop skills or experience which might be beneficial to your future career. If you are interested in academia, for example, you could get involved in a research project. Alternatively you could take this opportunity to explore specialised areas.

Intercalating

Students particularly interested in a topic related to medicine who want the opportunity to explore this in greater depth than is offered in the SSCs, may choose to take a year out of the medical programme to study an area in more detail. The timing of this will vary according to the medical school and in some medical schools you can take a BSc, MSc, MRes or MPhil depending again on how much of your course you have completed. Again, more details can be found in Chapter 8.

There is a wide range of subjects available for study in this manner. In addition to the usual subjects, such as anatomy, biochemistry and psychology, students may also undertake intercalated degrees in international health, health care ethics and public health. Further information on the range of intercalated degree options will be available from your medical school or at www.intercalate.co.uk.

Student exchange programme

Opportunities may also exist for students to spend a term or more studying at another European medical school under the Erasmus scheme. In terms of building your CV, taking part in Erasmus will give you the opportunity to demonstrate initiative, communication, organisational and planning skills as well as to gain experience in a different health care system.

Making the most of your clinical placements

Your clinical placements are an ideal way to develop and demonstrate the skills recruiters seek (see Chapter 10). They also provide you with the opportunity to build contacts and networks and to find out more about different areas of medicine. It is worth thinking about your placements in a critical manner to help form ideas about what you enjoy and are good at, what you don't enjoy, skills which you need to work on and develop, how you want to spend your future career and ways in which you can gain the skills, experience and knowledge which you will need in order to progress in different specialties.

ACTIVITY 11.4

- Find out as much as you can about the different specialties you come into contact with during your attachments.
- Talk to your consultant/GP supervisor. Ask about their specialty, what the work involves, good and bad aspects of their role, skill and academic entry requirements and training prior to registration.
- Talk to junior doctors who have recently gone through the application system and decision-making process to ask for helpful tips and advice.
- Make the most of your contacts. If you think you might want to pursue a career in radiology, ask the radiologist if you can spend some time with them.
- Get involved in any opportunities presented to take part in additional projects (e.g. helping with an audit or giving a presentation).
- Get involved in research initiatives. As well as developing your skills and experience you will be showing initiative, commitment and enthusiasm.

Teaching experience

Throughout your career as a doctor you will be teaching those less experienced than yourself so use any opportunity to develop some teaching skills. This experience will be looked on very favourably by selection panels. By the time you reach fourth and fifth years you will have gained many skills that you can pass on to others, so use any opportunities to develop your teaching skills whether to an individual or to small groups of students in the years below you.

Audit projects

These are covered in Chapter 8, but it is worth noting again that being a medical student gives you opportunities to carry out or become involved in an audit and also an opportunity to present the findings to other professionals which again will enhance your CV and make you stand out from your peers.

Medical school prizes

There are a number of these available, either locally within your medical school or nationally, and you should seek them out and not be afraid to apply for them. Internet searches in the area you are interested in can give you some ideas and your medical school may well have a list.

Published papers

Ideally, you could try to get your research from an intercalated degree or an SSC published in a peer-reviewed journal. Be prepared for a lot of work, as you may be asked to revise your work until they finally decide to publish it, or it may be rejected. If this is the case, don't give up. You could try to get it published in a non-indexed journal. Although these do not have the same impact as a peer-reviewed journal, they still make a good impression. You can try to get letters published in journals. You may also want to try and present at a conference or 'present' a poster. You could consider joining an organisation such as the Junior Association for the Study of Medical Education (JASME) (www.jasme.org.uk/index.html) if you are interested in research in any area of medical education.

Conclusion

You will not be able to get involved in all the activities outlined above but there will be some areas that you may be interested in which will develop your skills and experience and help you to get ahead of the competition. You will have to manage your own career within medicine so it follows that you need to be able to plan and develop the skills and experience that will make your CV stand out and develop personal attributes that will enable you to survive and thrive in the working environment. We hope this chapter has got you thinking on how you can start to progress your planning skills and develop your CV for that sought after specialty area.

Chapter summary

This chapter has:

- explained the importance of career planning;

- given you a structure to help plan for your future career;

- given you some activities to help you start to plan your career;

- described the different ways that you can start to build your CV for the future.

GOING FURTHER

- Cottrell, E (ed.) (2009) *The Medical Student Career Handbook*, 2nd revised edition. Oxford: Radcliffe Publishing.
  Written by medical students, this book provides information on the vast number of changes occurring in medical training.

- Elton, C and Reid, J (2007) *The Roads to Success: A Practical Approach to Career Planning for Medical Students, Foundation Trainees (and Their Supervisors)*. London: Postgraduate Deanery for Kent, Surrey, and Sussex.
  A useful introduction to career planning for medical students and foundation trainees.

- Riaz, A (2005) *Making Sense of Your Medical Career: Your Strategic Guide to Success*. London: Hodder Arnold.
  Lots of useful advice on how to make yourself more employable (written by a former medical student).

- Ward, C and Eccles, S (2001) *So You Want to be a Brain Surgeon? A Medical Careers Guide*. Oxford: Oxford University Press.
  Also new edition 2008, published by OUP as before and edited by Simon Eccles and Stephan Sanders. Breaks down what you need to know about getting into UK specialties and the training pathways required by the MMC.

chapter 12

Information Management

Dan Robinson

Achieving your medical degree

This chapter will help you to begin to meet the following requirements of *Tomorrow's Doctors* (GMC, 2009a):

Outcomes 2 – The doctor as a practitioner

19. Use information effectively in a medical context.

   (a) Keep accurate, legible and complete clinical records.
   (b) Make effective use of computers and other information systems, including storing and retrieving information.
   (c) Keep to the requirements of confidentiality and data protection legislation and codes of practice in all dealings with information.
   (d) Access information sources and use the information in relation to patient care, health promotion, giving advice and information to patients, and research and education.
   (e) Apply the principles, method and knowledge of health informatics to medical practice.

Chapter overview

By reading this chapter you will learn about the role that health informatics plays in the clinical setting. It will help you to understand the importance of being able to access, record and maintain information relating to health care.

Specifically you will learn about:

- the relationship between data information and knowledge;
- the role of health care records;
- data protection and legal issues;
- the importance of creating quality information;
- clinical systems and applications;
- essential information technology (IT) skills;
- e-portfolios and reflection.

Background

The management of health information, also referred to as 'health informatics', can be described as: 'The knowledge, skills and tools which enable information to be collected, managed, used and shared to support the delivery of health care and to promote health' (Department of Health, 2002).

It is recognised that informatics is now an integral part of clinical practice and supports key processes such as patient care, maintaining clinical records and professional competency. The data and information that is captured in each of these areas are interrelated and used for multiple purposes, such as providing knowledge to inform high-quality health care for the patient, assisting in clinical audit, resource planning and meeting current legal requirements.

The way in which data and information are created, maintained and communicated has changed dramatically in the last decade and the use of technology in the health care setting is playing an ever more pivotal role, with doctors now expected to use many different types of support systems which need specific skills and understanding. It is expected that all health care professionals need to have a good understanding of these various systems and the role that they play both at local and national level. As you progress in your medical career and move to postgraduate training, the knowledge you acquire will become ever more important. The skills which are required to use these systems are essential but it is also important that you understand the need for good-quality data and information, as this is at the core of good practice.

This chapter will outline the different types of information used in the clinical setting and the skills you will be able to develop as an undergraduate, before you start working as a doctor.

Understanding data, information and knowledge

To ensure high-quality patient care, it is vital that high-quality information is available at the appropriate time and with the appropriate person, in order to inform the decision-making process. This decision-making process is based on the knowledge and understanding of the doctor, which in turn is formed from information and data. Information is simply data which has been given a context.

Case study: Collecting information

Claire is a final-year medical student shadowing a junior doctor on a medical assessment unit late at night. She checks Mrs Smith's blood pressure, which is 130/80, and asks the doctor she is shadowing to put that down in the patient records on the end of her bed. She notices that earlier in the day her blood pressure was much higher at 160/90. She checks Mrs Smith's current drugs and previous treatment history on the computer in the nurses' station, which shows Mrs Smith is on a range of prescribed drugs at the moment. Both Claire and the doctor decide to keep a close eye on Mrs Smith's blood pressure for the rest of the night.

Knowledge is the collection of information in a form that is meaningful to the practitioner. This information is increasingly recorded electronically, using a variety of IT systems which you will become familiar with during your medical degree and clinical practice. The National Health Service (NHS) recognises that knowledge can be evidence based, derived from research, from statistical analysis of clinical data and also from experience.

In your role as a doctor you will need to ensure you have the necessary skills to access relevant sources of information and knowledge. You will then need to interpret and use this knowledge in relation to the needs of a service or patient to provide the best patient care (NHS, 2006).

Health care records

A health care record, or clinical care record, is defined by the Data Protection Act as 'any information relating to the physical or mental health or condition of an individual' that 'has been made by or on behalf of a health professional in connection with the care of that individual' (Department of Health, 2010).

Health records are stored in a number of different ways, which can be electronic or paper based. It is important that you understand how these are created, what they are used for and how they are stored. In recent years, clinical practice has had ever more reliance on how these records are stored electronically, how they are transferred and communicated in the clinical setting and beyond. The creation and communication of these electronic records often needs specialist skills and knowledge of numerous different software environments. As a student you will need to have the basic skills required to access these systems and will develop your knowledge and understanding as you progress to foundation training (see Chapter 10).

Health records serve two main functions, the most important of which is as a basis of information for doctors for clinical decision making and a means of communication between the doctor and patient. The second function is to act as a source of data which can then be analysed at local and national level, to provide a better standard of care through research, performance monitoring and service planning.

Patient access to information

Traditional models for the transferral of information from health care professionals to patients have taken the form of verbal communication in the health care setting.

With the advances in information technology, however, in particular the internet, there are now many portals of information by which the patient can access information about their own health care. Increasingly, patients are carrying out their own research before entering the clinical setting, which is then providing an environment where the patient can gain further understanding. Consequently, doctors now need to be aware of the various sources which patients may access before a clinical encounter, to effectively support patient communication (see Chapter 6).

The internet offers many different sources of information of varying quality and validity, but since much of the content is not regulated, caution should be used when accessing these sources. The NHS supports a number of sites offering good-quality up-to-date information. Some of the most accessed sites include:

- NHS Evidence Health Information Resources (formerly National Library for Health)
- NHS Clinical Knowledge Summaries – Information for patients
- NHS Choices
- Patient UK
- NHS Direct.

In addition to this, the NHS has introduced a Care Records Service which will allow both health care professionals and patients access to their own health records. For example, in England patients can access their Summary Care Record using the Health-Space secure website. As well as the central care record service, many GP surgeries are now offering patients access to their own health care records through projects such as EMIS (Egton Medical Information Systems Ltd), which is used by over 50 per cent of GP practices, and PAERS (Patient Access to Electronic Record Systems Ltd).

These are all examples of software solutions being developed in conjunction with the NHS but, in addition to this, there are also third-party sites which patients can now use to create their own record of health which can then be shared with their doctor, for example, Google Health and Microsoft Health Vault.

With so many sources of information surrounding medical conditions, and the ability for patients to access NHS records and create their own, it is important that you develop the knowledge and understanding of these various systems to provide the best-quality health care.

As a student, you will access health records under supervision. This will provide an opportunity to learn new skills and develop your understanding. You will also start to learn about patient confidentiality, which is covered later in this chapter.

ACTIVITY 12.1

You will already be familiar with some of the sources of information that patients can access, such as NHS Direct. Now search for a resource which you are not familiar with. Is this a creditable source of information? Would you recommend it as a source of information to a patient you come into contact with on a clinical placement?

Health care records – the future

As you progress through your medical degree it will be important for you to keep up to date with emerging technologies which will gradually play a more significant role in your education and future health care settings. Some of the new technologies you should be familiar with and understand how they are being used include:

- telehealth;

- web conferencing;

- virtual reality/patients;

- simulation;

- wireless information devices such as PDAs, laptops, tablets;

- web 2.0.

The last of these, web 2.0, is a term that has become popular in recent years and refers to web-based sites which allow users to easily create and share content, communicate and collaborate. You will be familiar with some of these sites such as social networking sites, blogs and video sharing sites, but they could also play an important role in future health care. For example:

- *The Personal Health Record (PHR); typically a health record that is initiated and maintained by an individual*

- *Personal Health Plans; the patient side of Pathways of Care that are currently paper-based*

- *Pathways of Care for Long Term Conditions; structured care plans tailored to individuals, encompassing social care, where care may be spread over many organisations and needs to be managed by the patient*

- *Patient empowerment; whereby patients work with their clinicians in partnership, to make their own choices and are able to act on them*

- *Communication; between the patient and Healthcare Professionals/care providers or between different Healthcare Professionals/care providers.*

(NHS Connecting for Health, 2009)

ACTIVITY 12.2

Find out more about Personal Health Records and think about the impact this may have on the patient–doctor clinical encounter and the treatment for the patient.

The health care record – your responsibilities

Good record keeping is the mark of the skilled and safe practitioner while careless or incompetent record keeping often highlights wider problems with the individual's practice.
(Nursing and Midwifery Council, 2005)

Information recorded in the clinical setting plays a critical role in clinical decision making and continuity of care. This is why your responsibility to gather and record high-quality data and information is so important. For example, as a junior doctor you could start a shift and have to make important decisions based on what has been written in patient records.

According to the GMC, doctors are expected to 'keep clear, accurate and legible records, reporting the relevant findings, the decisions made, the information given to patients, and any drugs prescribed or other investigation or treatment' and to 'make records at the same time as the events you are recording or as soon as possible afterwards' (GMC, 2010).

Each hospital will have their own specific guidelines on effective record keeping and it is important that you are aware of this document and its contents. Even though each hospital trust or primary care centre will have specific ways to create, maintain and communicate health records you will soon notice, as you become familiar with the different sources of these guidelines, that they are all based around a core set of recommendations.

The list below is a good practical guide published by the Medical Protection Society (2008) about creating good-quality clinical records.

- *Keeping good clinical records is essential for continuity of care, especially when many clinicians are involved in delivering care. Good record keeping is an integral part of good medical practice.*

- *Records should include sufficient detail for someone else to take over a patient's care, seamlessly, from where you left off.*

- *Records that secure continuity of care will also be adequate for evidential purposes, in the event of a complaint, claim or disciplinary action.*

- *Clinical records should be clear, objective, contemporaneous, tamper-proof and original.*

- *Abbreviations, if used, must be unambiguous and universally understood.*

- *Clinical records comprise handwritten and computerised notes, correspondence between health professionals, laboratory reports, x-ray and other imaging records, clinical photographs, videos and other recordings, and printouts from monitoring equipment.*

- *Clinical records are sensitive personal data and must be kept securely to prevent damage and unauthorised access.*

- *Clinical records can usually be shared with other members of the clinical teams responsible for clinical management, unless the patient objects.*

- *Access to records or the information they contain is also permissible in other circumstances but the record holder must always be prepared to justify disclosure.*

- *All health care organisations holding clinical records must be registered (under the Data Protection Act) with the Information Commissioner.*

- *Where information from clinical records is required for audit and research purposes, anonymised data should be used wherever possible.*

- *Records should not be kept indefinitely but should be retained as long as they are relevant to patient care and associated legal and administrative purposes.*

- *Any alteration to written medical records should be immediately apparent to avoid any accusation that there has been an attempt to mislead or deceive.*

- *Similarly, with electronic records, any entries should be made clear to identify any changes.*

- *Common problems are illegibility of handwritten notes, failing to date and sign them, inaccurate recording of information and insufficient detail.*

Other work in this field includes a collaboration between the Royal College of Physicians (2008) and NHS Connecting for Health (2009), who have developed standards for hospital patient records.

ACTIVITY 12.3

Locate the guidelines for good practice within the hospital nearest to your university. Is there anything specific to this policy which is in addition to the standard guidelines? Why do you think this may have been added?

Data protection and patient confidentiality

When dealing with patient information, there are clear ethical and legal obligations to ensure confidentiality. It is your responsibility to ensure that you fully understand these responsibilities and adhere to them both in your professional and personal life. Information disclosed to the doctor in confidence should not be disclosed in such a way which could lead to identification of the patient without their prior permission, and there can be severe consequences for those who do not adhere to this.

You will be expected to have an understanding of the relevant laws, guidelines and codes of practice. There are three primary areas:

- Department of Health's Confidentiality NHS Code of Practice;

- Caldicott Principles;

- Data Protection Act.

NHS Code of Practice: Confidentiality

The NHS Confidentiality Code of Practice is a comprehensive document which will help you to understand your responsibilities when using patient information. It gives useful background reading to the types of confidential patient information, how to provide a confidential service and how to make the correct decisions.

Caldicott Principles

The Caldicott Principles, which came out of the Caldicott Report of 1997 (Caldicott Committee, 1997) and relate to the safe management of patient-identifiable information, are the guidelines to which the NHS works. They cover information held in whatever format, whether paper based, electronic, verbal or visual, and should be adhered to whenever creating, maintaining or communicating patient-identifiable information.

The six principles are:

- Principle 1: Justify the purpose(s).
- Principle 2: Do not use personally identifiable information unless it is absolutely necessary.
- Principle 3: Use the minimum personally identifiable information.
- Principle 4: Access to personally identifiable information should be on a strict need to know basis.
- Principle 5: Everyone should be aware of their responsibilities.
- Principle 6: Understand and comply with the law.

The Data Protection Act

It is also important that you understand the basics of the Data Protection Act and how this relates to data in health care. You need to be aware, for example, that the Act applies to paper-based records and those stored electronically, and ensure that you abide by strict rules in terms of how patient information can be used and the rights of the patient to access this information.

What's the evidence?

The Data Protection Act 1984 was updated in 1998 and some important changes were made which reflected changes in society. Some of these changes were particularly relevant to health care. The following archived website highlights some important points in relation to health information management: http://webarchive. nationalarchives.gov.uk/+/www.dh.gov.uk/en/Managingyourorganisation/Informationpolicy/Recordsmanagement/DH_4000489

Knowledge bases, clinical systems and applications

So far, this chapter has covered some of the different types of information that you will be expected to access. However you will also need to have an understanding of different systems which store and manage information. As a student and then as a postgraduate you will need to understand the role, function and benefits of these systems at both local and national level. In addition to understanding the purpose of these you will also be expected to interact with them which will require specific IT skills.

A small example of systems you will be expected to use include:

- N3 – broadband networking services of the NHS;

- patient administration systems;

- clinical record systems;

- order communications (e.g. test requesting);

- scheduling systems (e.g. beds);

- GP2GP system;

- the electronic prescription service;

- the choose and book service.

In addition you will also need to understand the role and use of clinical knowledge and evidence-based resources and decision support systems, which are becoming ever increasingly used in clinical practice. Some examples of these are:

- NHS Evidence: Accesses a wide range of health information to help them deliver quality patient care.

- The NHS Clinical Knowledge Summaries (formerly PRODIGY): A reliable source of evidence-based information and practical 'know how' about the common conditions managed in primary care.

- National Electronic Library for Medicines (NeLM): The largest medicines information portal for health care professionals in the NHS. It aims to promote the safe, effective and efficient use of medicines.

- Map of Medicine: A visual representation of evidence-based, practice-informed care pathways. A knowledge resource that supports clinically led service improvement programmes, the Map has been shown to improve patient outcomes and lower health care delivery costs.

ACTIVITY 12.4

Find out more about the electronic support systems you will be expected to use during a community clinical placement. What type of information do these manage? Next time you look at a patient history, take note of the different types of information they contain relating to previous consultations in both hospital and community and previous drugs the patients have been prescribed. Speak to the practice manager about the issues surrounding maintaining patient confidentiality and patient records in a busy GP surgery.

Essential IT skills

Your university education and clinical practice will be supported by many different types of IT systems. Some of the clinical systems have already been covered in this chapter, but you will also have to interact with numerous other tools at university including:

- virtual learning environments;
- personal development planning tools;
- e-portfolios;
- clinical experience logging.

The IT skills which you develop during your undergraduate study will be invaluable throughout your career, with many of the skills being transferable across various systems, supporting many processes. For example, literature searching skills developed during your medical degree will support research when completing SSCs (see Chapter 8) or when studying for exams. Yet these valuable skills will also be used though your foundation training and beyond when completing various continuing professional development (CPD) activities and re-accreditation.

Utilising IT can also help you keep up to date with the latest treatments and debates within medicine when you are qualified as a doctor as you will not have time to read through every journal and every medical book.

Tomorrow's Doctors (GMC, 2009a, page 57) also requires you to maintain a portfolio of evidence of achievement and this is often supported during your undergraduate education and during foundation training by the use of an e-portfolio. Within education, e-portfolios are implemented to support a number of activities, usually for personal development planning, assessment recording and feedback, recording of clinical activity and feedback.

As you progress from undergraduate to foundation training you will understand the importance of keeping an e-portfolio. The information which you build during your time as a student will be useful when applying for foundation posts, when you will be asked for examples of specific experience. It is also a requirement to maintain an e-portfolio during your foundation training and is becoming more prevalent in supporting CPD activities of qualified doctors. You will also find as you maintain a portfolio of achievement and previous experience that you will develop your reflective practice skills, which are often assessed in undergraduate education (see Chapter 5).

Case study: IT skills

Jayne is a student at the University of Liverpool. Towards the end of the first year she has to attend a 'feedback appraisal' where she has the opportunity to discuss her first year with her problem-based learning (PBL) tutors. As part of this process there are a number of pieces of evidence which need to be presented.

This evidence has been gathered throughout the year, using various electronic systems, including:

- VITAL (Virtual Interactive Teaching and Learning at Liverpool) which is a virtual learning environment (VLE) and hosts activities such as 'The consideration of an ethical issue', whereby Jayne is asked to comment on appropriate action of a given scenario;
- LUSID: an online personal development planning (PDP) support tool where Jayne has to reflect on her performance in her formative exams;
- feedback from clinical log books on performance during the year.

Before her appraisal, Jayne is able to access this evidence and present it to her PBL tutor to demonstrate her progress during the year. As Jayne progresses through her undergraduate years, she keeps a comprehensive e-portfolio of academic achievements, key clinical experiences and reflective practice which she then uses to support her application for foundation training.

When Jayne starts her foundation doctor training she is expected to maintain an NHS e-portfolio. The skills she has developed over her undergraduate years play an important role in maintaining this important record and helped in her application for specialist training.

As an undergraduate you will have many opportunities to develop your IT skills. Your university will offer training courses to enable you to use the various electronic systems which will be available to you. Ask at your university library for more information. If you feel you need more than basic training you can complete something like the European Computer Driving Licence, which covers topics such as the use of word processing, spreadsheets and databases which will be useful for your undergraduate studies and beyond.

For example:

- NHS ELITE (NHS eLearning IT Essentials) covers essential IT skills, such as how to use a keyboard and mouse through to file management, web and email skills.

- NHS Health (NHS eLearning for Health Information Systems) covers essential information to ensure users comply with information governance, data protection and patient confidentiality requirements (NHS Connecting for Health, 2009, page 11).

Maintaining IT skills as you progress through your career will be as important a part of your clinical practice as treating your patients and will help you treat your patients in the future, so having a qualification in IT could help you to become a better doctor.

Chapter summary

This chapter has:

- demonstrated the importance of good-quality data and how this relates to providing quality health care;

- highlighted how health care records are created, maintained and used;

- described the importance of patient confidentiality;

- given an overview of clinical systems and applications and the IT skills you will need to use these effectively;

- shown that IT skills are essential for doctors and students.

GOING FURTHER

- Department of Health (2003) *Confidentiality: NHS Code of Practice.* www. dh.gov.uk/en/Publicationsandstatistics/Publications/PublicationsPolicy-AndGuidance/DH_4069253 (accessed February 2011).
  A good reference source if you wanted clarification on a specific issue.

- Department of Health (2010) Patient confidentiality and access to health records. www.dh.gov.uk/en/Managingyourorganisation/Informationpolicy/Patientconfidentialityandcaldicottguardians/index.htm (accessed February 2011).
  A good mini-site hosted by the Department of Health on many of the issues covered in this chapter.

- NHS Connecting for Health (2011a) Essential IT Skills (EITS). www.connectingforhealth.nhs.uk/systemsandservices/etd/eits (accessed February 2011).
  Further information on the essential IT skills you will be required to attain, including links to NHS Elite, NHS Health and ECDL.

- NHS Connecting for Health (2011b) Acronyms guide: learn what ours mean. www.connectingforhealth.nhs.uk/factsandfiction/acronyms (accessed February 2011).
  A very useful reference site of acronyms and links to further information.

- Royal College of Physicians (2008) *A Clinician's Guide to Record Standards.* www.rcplondon.ac.uk/clinical-standards/hiu/medical-records/Pages/Overview.aspx (accessed February 2011).
  A comprehensive guide on medical record keeping and what you can do to ensure good practice.

chapter 13

Future Directions in Medical Education
Simon Watmough

Achieving your medical degree

The final paragraph of the introduction to *Tomorrow's Doctors* (GMC, 2009a, page 7) states:

> *Today's undergraduates – tomorrow's doctors – will see huge changes in medical practice. There will be continuing developments in biomedical sciences and clinical practice, new health priorities, rising expectations among patients and the public and changing societal attitudes. Basic knowledge and skills, while fundamentally important, will not be enough on their own. Medical students must be inspired to learn about medicine in all its future aspects so as to serve patients and become doctors of the future. With that perspective and commitment, allied to specific knowledge, skills and behaviours set out in* Tomorrow's Doctors and Good Medical Practice, *they will be well placed to provide and to improve the health and care of patients, as scholars and scientists, practitioners and professionals.*

Introduction

This book has introduced to you some of the key themes which run through *Tomorrow's Doctors* and undergraduate medical education in the UK. It does not go into detail about every aspect of *Tomorrow's Doctors* or indeed every aspect of medical education, but we hope it has drawn your attention to some themes which you may have been unaware of. We hope you will enjoy the activities and scenarios and will use the references and 'What's the evidence' sections to explore these areas further. We also hope you will take the opportunity to read through *Tomorrow's Doctors* and explore on your own any areas which interest you. As has been highlighted throughout this book – particularly the SSC chapter – exploring areas which interest you is a key skill to develop for any medical student and doctor.

The General Medical Council's (GMC's) place in undergraduate medical education in the UK is often misunderstood or simply not known about and Chapters 1 and 2 have tried to clarify the role and influence of the GMC on medical education. These chapters have also explained some of the other influences on undergraduate medical education in the UK and why your undergraduate course looks like it does. We hope that this book has shown that medical curricula look the way they do for a reason and there is more to being a good doctor than just learning about diseases and sciences.

We also hope we have helped to show that what you learn as an undergraduate is geared towards making you as good a doctor as it is possible for you to be and there are lots of opportunities as an undergraduate to prepare yourself for working as a doctor and learning to manage your career.

ACTIVITY 13.1

This book has highlighted a number of key documents, from the GMC and from other bodies which have directly influenced medical education in the UK. Count how many have been mentioned in this book. Do you think they are all as important as each other?

ACTIVITY 13.2

Research another area of *Tomorrow's Doctors* that interests you that hasn't been covered in this book. Think about why it is included in *Tomorrow's Doctors*, how you might experience that as an undergraduate and how it will benefit you working as a doctor.

Future directions in medical education

This section will briefly summarise how medical education might develop in the next few years in general and make specific reference to the topics covered in this book. In the UK two books have speculated about how medical education in the UK might develop in the future (Calman, 2006; Bleakley *et al.*, 2011). There has also been speculation outside the UK about how medical education might develop; for example, the Association of Faculties of Medicine of Canada in 2010 published a document entitled *The Future of Medical Education in Canada: A Collective Vision for MD Education*. The key word here is 'might' as no one can accurately predict the future and pretending you can is one way to make yourself look stupid! Few people in the 1980s would have predicted the impact the internet would have on the world we live in today. Many people were surprised by the content of the first *Tomorrow's Doctors* when it was published as well. However, it is possible to speculate by looking at trends in medical education since 1993.

Some of the reasons for the original publication of *Tomorrow's Doctors* have not changed. For example, the growth of scientific knowledge and therefore potential overcrowding in the curriculum has continued, improvements in IT have accelerated and the public's expectations of the professionalism they expect from a doctor has not diminished. In fact it could be argued, given the explosion in the use of the internet and the growth of 24-hour media coverage since 1993 and some of the scandals surrounding the medical profession such as the Harold Shipman case, that patients' expectations of their doctors regarding professionalism have increased exponentially.

Although it is not possible to say exactly how medical education will evolve for certain, it is extremely unlikely that medical curricula will revert to how they were before the first edition of *Tomorrow's Doctors*. For example, despite the fact there may be more emphasis on some of the sciences as outlined in Chapters 1 and 2, there is unlikely to be a return to traditional courses with two years of preclinical lectures without any early specific clinical skills training, for example. Also, it is inconceivable that medical schools will be able to run an undergraduate course without any communication skills tuition in the future, even if they wanted to.

If there is not an updated *Tomorrow's Doctors* while you are at medical school, there almost certainly will be while you are working as a doctor. This will impact on how you teach and supervise students. There will probably be updated guidance from other bodies with an influence on medical education such as the European Union and the UK Royal Colleges, for example. Chapters 1 and 2 have explained how regulation of medical education in the UK has evolved. It will continue to evolve in the future and it is inconceivable that there will be a return to the situation before 1858 with no regulation of medicine/medical education. In the extremely unlikely event of the GMC being disbanded then another regulatory body would take its place.

Since 1993 the GMC has brought out many documents on undergraduate and postgraduate medical education and on the skills and attributes it expects fully qualified doctors to possess. Although many have been updated since they were first published, the subsequent documents have built on themes contained in the previous documents and this is likely to continue while responding to any unforeseen developments either in medicine or changes in society.

As stated above, the expectations of the regulatory bodies and public regarding professionalism of medical students and doctors will not change and you will still be expected to behave like a professional, and if anything these expectations may intensify. A new version of *Good Medical Practice: Duties of a Doctor* is in consultation at the time of writing; this will show the standards expected of you when you work as a doctor. Good communication skills are intrinsically linked to professionalism. In recent years, poor communication skills have been the reason for the highest number of complaints about doctors in the UK, so communication skills will not diminish in importance.

For communication skills training it is likely that technology will continue to be utilised. Simulation could see the quickest developments as technology improves. This could mean changes to clinical skills and anatomy resource centres in both universities and hospitals. Surgeons of the future will find the options for simulated training increasing once they have graduated. Like simulation, informatics is to continue to become an increasingly important part of medical education and medicine. It is likely patients' records will all be held on electronic databases and there will be an increased use of podcasts and the internet for teaching.

Recording your achievements and the development of your skills as an undergraduate and postgraduate will increasingly take place through electronic portfolios. These will also be used for evidence when applying for postgraduate positions and monitoring continuing professional development. At the same time, more and more journal articles will be restricted to internet publication only and more books will be available for downloading to electronic devices.

Previously, assessment for medical students largely consisted of written examinations; Chapter 5 has shown how far assessment has developed in recent years. While there will always be a written component to both undergraduate (and postgraduate) exams, assessments will continue to use a variety of methods. Recently, consultant and GP appraisals were introduced for senior doctors and it is likely this will evolve until all doctors are continually assessed throughout their working lives. This will also mean that the ability to give and receive peer feedback will remain essential for all doctors.

A national prescribing test is likely be introduced for all students in the UK in the next couple of years and there is a debate about a national licensing exam for medical students in the UK, which is an 'exit' exam for graduates, based on existing systems in North America which all students from all universities would be required to pass prior to working as a doctor. An exit exam, if implemented, would drive assessment change in undergraduate medical curricula and could also change how medical students view their undergraduate education. It could also change how GMC guidelines are interpreted by medical schools in their undergraduate courses as all medical schools will want their graduates to perform well in a licensing exam.

Student selected components will continue to vary across different medical schools while retaining the key features outlined in Chapter 8 and the skills and opportunities they provide to medical students will continue to be important. As already stated, clinical knowledge will continue to increase so students will need options to explore areas not covered in the 'core curriculum' and learn essential research skills. Clinical attachments will continue to be the place where students practise diagnosing, examining, treating, talking to patients, learn practical skills and receive the opportunity to prepare themselves for being a doctor. The emphasis has been on using these to prepare students for working as a doctor either through shadowing or now assistantships – these could be developed so that students have even more supervised experiences of undertaking the role of a foundation doctor before they begin work.

Three universities in the UK (Liverpool, Dundee and Glasgow) have at the time of writing final exams before the end of the final year to allow students to practise working as a junior doctor without the pressure of final examinations. More medical schools may move towards this model. Although the doctor's role as a leader has shifted within the multidisciplinary team (as highlighted in Chapter 4), doctors will still be responsible for leading teams, supervising medical students and junior doctors and setting the example for future generations of doctors. The ethos of team working in the NHS is also very unlikely to diminish in future years.

Not many students graduating in the years after 2000 would have predicted the Modernising Medical Careers (MMC) reforms and although a major shake-up of training on that scale may not be imminent, competition for training posts will remain fierce in the coming years. Being prepared to manage your career will clearly become even more important.

Recently, a document issued by the Medical Schools Council, which has included consultation with foundation schools, consultants, the GMC, Department of Health and the British Medical Association (BMA) among others, has suggested that there should be a standardised scheme for medical schools to grade students' clinical knowledge and skills based on a student's performance to date. Instead of 'white spaced questions' on the foundation application form there will be an invigilated 'machine-markable' [sic] test of professional attributes similar to the tests for GP training. It is proposed that students would take a Situational Judgement Test (Medical Schools Council, 2010) which will ask them to choose from a range of options how they would respond to a series of real life clinical situations. At the time of writing these are now being piloted, possibly to be introduced in the near future. This highlights the fact that innovations in medicine and medical education are always likely despite the fact MMC is still relatively new – and there are working parties thinking about ways of changing (and hopefully improving) the status quo in medical education.

What's the evidence?

The introduction of a licensing exam along the lines of exams already taken in North America would have a major impact on undergraduate medical education in the UK.

The following articles in the *Student BMJ* written by students show arguments for and against a national licensing exam. They can be accessed via the archive: Should UK medical students sit a national licensing exam? Available from http://archive.student.bmj.com/issues/08/05/life/184.php (accessed 6 December 2010):

- Kelly, C (2008) Yes. *Student BMJ*, 16: 184.
- Burke, K (2008) No. *Student BMJ*, 16: 185.

Other articles arguing for and against a national licensing exam include:

- Harden, R. (2009) Five myths and the case against a European or national licensing examination. *Medical Teacher*, 31(3): 217–220.
- Schuwirth, L (2007) The need for national licensing examinations. *Medical Education*, 41: 1022–1023.

ACTIVITY 13.3

The GMC consults widely before issuing updated recommendations. They advertise their consultations on their website. Next time they undertake a consultation exercise, consider contributing to this process to help future cohorts of students and the doctors you will be working with in the future.

Conclusion

Studying for a medical degree is hard work, but being a medical student and then a doctor can be immensely rewarding and enjoyable. Medical education is an evolutionary process, which reflects the changing expectations of patients and society. Regulatory bodies must also continue to assist medical schools to develop their undergraduate curricula to reflect these expectations. This book has aimed to provide the first step towards your awareness of developments in medical education and to show you that there may be more to your medical degree and career than you previously thought. There are many ways as an undergraduate to keep in touch with any future changes or reforms. In addition to publications by the GMC, the NHS and the Royal Colleges, university websites, broadsheet newspapers and organisations such as the BBC will often report issues related to medicine and medical education. Making sure you are aware of any future changes will help you to meet the challenges of studying as an undergraduate and working as a doctor and help you to become better prepared to treat your patients.

Chapter summary

- Medical education will continue to evolve.

- It is impossible to say exactly which direction it will take, although it is possible to speculate about some changes.

- Being aware of these changes could help you become a better doctor.

GOING FURTHER

- Association of Faculties of Medicine of Canada (2010) *The Future of Medical Education in Canada: A Collective Vision for MD Education*. Available from: www.afmc.ca/fmec/pdf/collective_vision.pdf (accessed 6 December 2010). *This paper speculates about the future of medical education in Canada.*

- Bleakley, A, Bligh, J and Brice, J (2011) *Medical Education for the Future: Identity, Power and Location* (Advances in Medical Education). Heidelberg: Springer.
This book speculates about the future of medical education in the UK.

References

Albanese, M and Mitchell, S (1993) Problem-based learning: a review of literature on its outcomes and implementation issues. *Academic Medicine*, 68: 52–81.

Arnold, L and Stern, DT (2006) What is medical professionalism? in Stern, DT (ed.) *Measuring Medical Professionalism*. Oxford: Oxford University Press, pp. 15–38.

Association of Faculties of Medicine of Canada (2010) *The Future of Medical Education in Canada: A Collective Vision for MD Education*. www.afmc.ca/fmec/pdf/collective_vision.pdf (accessed 6 December 2010).

Bleakley, A, Bligh, J and Brice, J (2011) *Medical Education for the Future: Identity, Power and Location* (Advances in Medical Education Series). Berlin: Springer.

Brennan, N, Corrigan, O and Allard, J (2010) The transition from medical student: today's experiences of *Tomorrow's Doctors*. *Medical Education*, 44: 449–458.

Bullimore, D (1998) *Study Skills and Tomorrow's Doctors*. London: WB Saunders.

Caldicott Committee (1997) *The Caldicott Report*. Department of Health. http://confidential.oxfordradcliffe.net/caldicott/report (accessed February 2011).

Calman, K (2006) *Medical Education: Past, Present and Future: Handing on Learning*. London: Churchill Livingstone.

Calman, K and Donaldson, M (1991) The pre-registration house officer year: a critical incident study. *Medical Education*, 25: 51–59.

Centre for Change and Innovation (2003) *Talking Matters: Developing the Communication Skills of Doctors*. Edinburgh: Scottish Executive.

Chartered Society of Physiotherapy (2000) *General Principles of Good Record Keeping and Access to Health Records*. www.csp.org.uk/uploads/documents/csp_physioprac_pa47.pdf (accessed February 2011).

Chief Medical Officer (2009) *Safer Medical Practice: Machines, Manikins and Polo Mints. 150 Years of the Annual Report of the Chief Medical Officer: On the State of Public Health 2008*. London: Department of Health.

Chipp, E, Stoneley, S and Cooper, K (2004) Clinical placements for medical students: factors affecting patients' involvement in medical education. *Medical Teacher*, 26(2): 114–119.

Cleland, JA, Milne, A, Sinclair, H and Lee, AJ (2009) An intercalated degree is associated with higher marks in subsequent medical school examinations. *BMC Medical Education*, 9: 24.

Clinical Skills Managed Educational Network (2009) *Pilot of the Mobile Clinical Skills Unit: Evaluation of the First Six Months*. www.csmen.ac.uk/projects/documents/Reporton1st6monthsofMobileUnitPilot.pdf (accessed February 2011).

Cusimano, MD (1996) Standard setting in medical education. *Academic Medicine*, 71: S112–S120.

Darzi, A (2008) *High Quality Care for All: NHS Next Stage Review Final Report*. CM 7432. London: Department of Health.

Dennison, B and Kirk, R (1990) *Do, Review, Learn, Apply*. Oxford: Blackwell.

Department of Health (2002) *Making Information Count: A Human Resources Strategy for Health Informatics Professionals*. www.dh.gov.uk/prod_consum_dh/groups/dh_digitalassets/@dh/@en/documents/digitalasset/dh_4073084.pdf (accessed February 2011).

Department of Health (2003) *Guiding Principles Relating to the Commissioning and Provision of Communication Skills Training in Preregistration and Undergraduate Education for Healthcare Professionals*. London: Department of Health.

Department of Health (2005) *NHS Modernising Medical Careers Working Group for Career Management. Career Management: An Approach for Medical Schools, Deaneries, Royal Colleges and Trusts*. London: Department of Health.

Department of Health (2010) *Confidentiality*. www.dh.gov.uk/en/Publicationsandstatistics/Publications/PublicationsPolicyAndGuidance/Browsable/DH_5133529 (accessed February 2011).

Dismukes, RK, Gaba, DM and Howard, SK (2006) So many roads: facilitated debriefing in healthcare. *Simulation in Healthcare*, 1: 23–26.

Elliott, DD, May, W, Schaff, PB, Nyquist, JG, Trial, J, Reilly, JM and Lattore, P (2009) Shaping professionalism in pre clinical medical students: professionalism and the practice of medicine. *Medical Teacher*, 31: e295–e302.

Fraser, R (1991) Undergraduate medical education: present state and future needs. *British Medical Journal*, 303: 41–43.

Fried, G, Feldman, L, Vassiliou, M, Fraser, S, Stanbridge, D, Ghitulescu, G and Andrew, C (2004) Proving the value of simulation in laparoscopic surgery. *Annals of Surgery*, 240: 518.

Gaba, DM (2004) The future vision of simulation in health care. *Quality and Safety in Health Care*, 13: i2–i10.

Garner, J, McKendree, J, O'Sullivan, H and Taylor, D (2010) Undergraduate medical student attitudes to the peer assessment of professional behaviours in two medical schools. *Education for Primary Care*, 21: 32–37.

GMC (General Medical Council) (1957) *Tomorrow's Doctors: Recommendations as to the Medical Curriculum*. London: General Medical Council.

References

GMC (1993) *Tomorrow's Doctors: Recommendations on Undergraduate Medical Education*. London: GMC.

GMC (1997) *The New Doctor*. London: GMC.

GMC (2006, updated March 2009) *Good Medical Practice*. London: GMC.

GMC (2009a) *Tomorrow's Doctors*. London: GMC.

GMC (2009b) *Medical Students: Professional Values and Fitness to Practise*. London: GMC. www.gmc-uk.org/static/documents/content/Medical_Students_-_professional_values_and_fitness_to_practice_Oct_2010.pdf (accessed February 2011).

GMC (2010) *Good Medical Practice*. www.gmc-uk.org/guidance/good_medical_practice/contents.asp (accessed February 2011).

Goodenough, W (1944) Great Britain, Ministry of Health and Department of Health for Scotland. *Report of the Inter-departmental Committee on Medical Schools*. (Chairman: Sir William Goodenough). London: HMSO.

Gordon, J, Wilkerson, W, Shaffer, D and Armstrong, E (2001) 'Practicing' medicine without risk: students' and educators' responses to high-fidelity patient simulation. *Academic Medicine*, 76: 469–472.

Hafferty, F (1998) Beyond curriculum reform: confronting medicine's hidden curriculum. *Academic Medicine*, 73: 403–407.

Halperin, E (2000) Grievances against physicians: 11 years experience of a medical society grievance committee. *Western Journal of Medicine*, 173: 235–238.

Hargie, O, Boohan, M, McCoy, M and Murphy, P (2010) Current trends in communication skills training in UK schools of medicine. *Medical Teacher* 32(5): 385–391.

Hendrickx, K, De Winter, B, Wyndaele, J, Tjalma, W, Debaene, L, Selleslags, B, Mast, F, Buytaert, P and Bossaert, L (2006) Intimate examination teaching with volunteers: implementation and assessment at the University of Antwerp. *Patient Education and Counseling*, 63: 47–54.

Hofstee, WKB (1983) The case for compromise in educational selection and grading, in Anderson, SN and Helmick, JS (eds) *On Educational Testing*. San Francisco: Jossey-Bass.

Howe, A, Barrett, A and Leinster, S (2009) How medical students demonstrate their professionalism when reflecting on experience. *Medical Education*, 43: 942–951.

Illing, J, Peile, E and Morrison, J and others (2008) *How Prepared Are Medical Graduates to Begin Practice? A Comparison of Three Diverse Medical Schools*. Final Report for the GMC Education Committee. London: GMC.

Irvine, D (1993) General practice in the 1990s: a personal view on future developments. *British Journal of General Practice*, 43: 121–125.

Kneebone, R, Arora, S, King, D, Bello, F, Sevdalis, N, Kassab, E, AggarwaL, R, Darzi,

A and Nestel, D (2010) Distributed simulation – accessible immersive training. *Medical Teacher*, 32: 65–70.

Laidlaw, A and Hart, J (2011). Communication skills: an essential component of medical curricula. Part I: Assessment of clinical communication: AMEE Guide No. 511. *Medical Teacher*, 33: 6–8.

Levenson, R, Atkinson, S and Shepherd, S (2010) *The 21st Century Doctor: Understanding the Doctors of Tomorrow*. London: The Kings Fund. www.kingsfund.org.uk/current_projects/the_21stcentury_doctor/ (accessed February 2011).

Medical Protection Society (2008) MPS guide to medical records. www.medicalprotection.org/uk/booklets/MPS-guide-to-medical-records (accessed February 2011).

Medical Schools Council (2010) Improving selection to the Foundation Programme. www.medschools.ac.uk/AboutUs/Projects/isfp/Pages/default.aspx (accessed 6 December 2010).

Merrison Report (1975) *Report of the Committee of Inquiry into the Regulation of the Medical Profession*, Cmnd. 6018. London: HMSO.

Miller, GE (1990) The assessment of clinical skills/competence/performance. *Academic Medicine*, 65: S63–S67.

Murdoch-Eaton, D, Ellershaw, J, Garden, A, Newble, D, Perry, M, Robinson, L, Smith, J, Stark, P and Whittle, S (2004) Student-selected components in the undergraduate medical curriculum: a multi-institutional consensus on purpose. *Medical Teacher*, 26: 33–38.

Murphy, J, De Senaviratne, R, Remers, O and Davis, M (2009) Student selected components: student-designed modules are associated with closer alignment of planned and learned outcomes. *Medical Teacher*, 31: 489–483.

Naik, V, Matsumoto, E, Houston, P, Hamstra, S, Yeung, R, Mallon, J and Martire, T (2001) Fiberoptic orotracheal intubation on anesthetized patients: do manipulation skills learned on a simple model transfer into the operating room? *Anesthesiology*, 95: 343.

Newble, D (1998) Assessment, in Jolly, B and Rees, C (eds) *Medical Education in the New Millennium*. Oxford: Oxford University Press, pp. 131–142.

NHS (2006) National Knowledge Service. www.nks.nhs.uk/bestcurrentknowledge.asp (accessed February 2011).

NHS (2010) *NHS White Paper, Equity and Excellence: Liberating the NHS*. London: NHS.

NHS Connecting for Health (2009) *Learning to Manage Health Information: A Theme for Clinical Education*. www.connectingforhealth.nhs.uk/systemsandservices/capability/health/hidcurriculum/brochure.pdf (accessed February 2011).

Norcini, J, Blank, L, Arnold, G and Kimball, H (1995) The Mini-CEX (Clinical

Evaluation Exercise): a preliminary investigation. *Annals of Internal Medicine*, 123: 795–799.

Nursing and Midwifery Council (2005) *Guidelines for Records and Record Keeping*. London: NMC.

Papadakis, MA, Teherani, A, Banach, MA, Knettler, TR, Rattner, SL, Stern, DT, Veloski, JJ and Hodgson, CS (2005) Disciplinary action by medical boards and prior behaviour in medical school. *New England Journal of Medicine*, 353(25): 2673–2682.

Parsell, G and Bligh, J (1995) The changing context of undergraduate medical education. *Postgraduate Medical Journal*, 71: 394–403.

Perrera, J, Mohamodu, G and Kaur, S (2010) The use of objective structured self-assessment and peer-feedback (OSSP) for learning communication skills: evaluation using a controlled trial. *Advances in Health Sciences Education*, 15: 185–193.

Porritt, A (1962) *A Review of the Medical Services in Great Britain: Report of the Medical Services Review Committee (the Porritt Report)*. London: Social Assay.

Poynter, F (1966) *The Evolution of Medical Education in Britain*. London: Pitman Medical Publishing.

QAA (Quality Assurance Agency for Higher Education) (2000). Subject overview report, Medicine. www.qaa.ac.uk/academicinfrastructure/benchmark/honours/medicine.asp (accessed February 2011).

Ramani, S and Leinster, S (2008) AMEE Guide no. 34: Teaching in the clinical environment. *Medical Teacher*, 30(4): 347–364.

Royal College of Physicians (2005) *Doctors in Society: Medical Professionalism in a Changing World*. London: RCP.

Royal College of Physicians (2008) Medical record keeping. www.rcplondon.ac.uk/clinical-standards/hiu/medical-records/Pages/Overview.aspx (accessed February 2011).

Royal College of Physicians (2009) *Trust in Doctors 2009: Annual Survey of Public Trust in Professions*. London: RCP.

Riley, S (2009) Student Selected Components (SSCs): AMEE Guide no. 46. *Medical Teacher*, 31: 885–894.

Schonrock-Adema, J, Heijne-Penninga, M, van Duijn, MAJ, Geertsma, J and Cohen-Schotanus, J (2007) Assessment of professional behaviour in undergraduate medical education: peer assessment enhances performance. *Medical Education*, 41: 836–842.

Shacklady, J, Holmes, E, Mason, G, Davies, I and Dornan, T (2009) Maturity and medical students' ease of transition into the clinical environment. *Medical Teacher*, 31(7): 621–626.

Shumway, J and Harden, R (2003) AMEE Guide N0.25: The assessment of learning outcomes for the competent and reflective physician. *Medical Teacher*, 25, 569–584

Skills for Health (2009) *Junior Doctors in the NHS: Preparing Medical Students for*

Employment and Postgraduate Training. www.skillsforhealth.org.uk/~/media/
Resource-Library/PDF/Tomorrows-Doctors-2009.ashx (accessed 22 October 2010).

Stacey, M (1992) *Regulating British Medicine. The General Medical Council.* Chichester:
John Wiley & Sons.

Tooke, J (2008) *Aspiring to Excellence. Findings and Final Recommendations of the
Independent Inquiry into Modernising Medical Careers.* Aldridge Press: London.
www.mmcinquiry.org.uk/Final_8_Jan_08_MMC_all.pdf (accessed February 2011).

University of Liverpool (2010) *MBChB Generic Programme Handbook 2010–11.*
http://www.liv.ac.uk/sme/administration/Generic%20Handbook%202010-
11FINAL.pdf (accessed February 2011).

University of Sheffield (2010) Student selected components. www.sheffield.ac.uk/
aume/curriculum_dev/ssc.html (accessed February 2011).

Warren, P and Parnell, M (2011) Medical leadership: why it is important, what is
required and how we develop it. *Postgraduate Medical Journal*, 87: 27–32.

Wass, V and Van Der Vleuten, C (2004) The long case. *Medical Education*, 38:
1176–1180.

Wass, V, Van Der Vleuten, C, Shatzer, J and Jones, R (2001) Assessment of clinical
competence. *The Lancet*, 357: 945–949.

Watmough, S, Waddelove, C and Jaeger, L (2009) First year medical students'
perceptions of a career in medicine – how can these inform careers support? in
Constructing the Future: Career Guidance for Changing Contexts. Stourbridge: Institute
of Career Guidance.

Watzlawick, P, Beavin-Bavelas, J and Jackson, D (1967) *Some Tentative Axioms of
Communication. Pragmatics of Human Communication – A Study of Interactional
Patterns, Pathologies and Paradoxes.* New York: WW Norton.

Weller, J (2004) Simulation in undergraduate medical education: bridging the gap
between theory and practice. *Medical Education*, 38: 32–38.

WFME (World Federation for Medical Education) (2003) *Basic Medical Education:
WFME Global Standards for Quality Improvement.* www.wfme.org (accessed February
2011).

Whitehouse, A, Hassell, A, Wood, L, Wall, D, Walzman, M and Campbell, I (2005)
Development and reliability testing of TAB a form for 360 degree assessment of
Senior House Officers' professional behaviour, as specified by the General Medical
Council. *Medical Teacher*, 27: 252–258.

Williams, G and Lau, A (2004) Reform of undergraduate medical teaching in the
United Kingdom: a triumph of evangelism over common sense. *British Medical
Journal*, 329: 92.

Wilson, M (2004) *The Medic's Guide to Work and Electives around the World.* London:
Arnold.

Index